Table of Contents

Coping
A Practical Guide for People with Life-Challenging Diseases and their Caregivers

Rubin Battino, M.S.
Mental Health Counseling, Adjunct Professor,
Department of Human Services (Counseling)
Wright State University

Illustrations by Mario Uribe

Crown House Publishing
www.crownhouse.co.uk

First published in the UK by

Crown House Publishing Limited
Crown Buildings
Bancyfelin
Carmarthen
Wales
SA33 5ND
UK

www.crownhouse.co.uk

Permission to quote from the following source is gratefully
acknowledged: Oldways Preservation & Exchange Trust for the Traditional
Mediterranean diet pyramid.

The author would like to acknowledge the following: JOSSEY-BASS INC.,
PUBLISHERS to excerpt from *Living With Life-Threatening Illness* by Kenneth J.
Doka; G.P. PUTNAM'S SONS to excerpt from *The Wellness Community Guide to
Fighting for Recovery from Cancer* by Harold H. Benjamin; HARPER & ROW to
excerpt from *Love, Medicine and Miracles* by Bernie Siegel; PENGUIN BOOKS USA
INC. to excerpt from *Giving Comfort* by Linda Breiner Milstein and *Cancer as a
Turning Point* by Lawrence LeShan. The author's failure to obtain permission for
the use of any other copyrighted material included in this work is inadvertent
and will be corrected in future printings of the work.

British Library of Cataloguing-in-Publication Data
A catalogue entry for this book is available from the British Library.

ISBN 1899836683

Typeset by Mac Style, Scarborough, N. Yorkshire
Printed and bound in Wales by
Gomer Press
Llandysul

Dedication

This book is dedicated to my
friend Carol E. Dixon for her help
in shaping this book, her years of
service to Hospice of Dayton,
and simply for her friendship.

Preface

At last night's meeting of our exceptional patient support group there were three new members: a man in his late sixties with a recent diagnosis of cancer, his wife of over forty years, and one of his sons. Attending the support group was just one of the many things Sam (not his real name) and his family are doing. They are seeking second and third opinions at major cancer centers, and they have begun the arduous search for information on his particular cancer. What else can Sam and his wife and family do? Fortunately, at this stage, Sam's attitude is upbeat and hopeful. Feeling hopeful enhances the body's capacity to fight disease. Feeling hopeless and helpless and out of control diminishes this capacity. This book is a compendium of the many ways you can cope (rhymes with hope!) with a diagnosis of, living with, and fighting a life-challenging disease. There are many things that Sam and his caregivers can do to face this challenge. The Viennese psychiatrist Viktor E. Frankl has pointed out that we have no control over what challenges life may present us, but we always have the choice of *how* we will respond. This book is also about choice.

The introductory chapter covers some material about the words we use, like useful distinctions between disease and illness, and also between curing and healing. The scientific evidence for attitude being helpful, as manifested in David Spiegel's work on support groups, provides the basis for recommending the many varieties of coping discussed later in the book. Relaxation has been shown to enhance the body's defenses—Chapter Two is about several relaxation methods. This chapter ends with a few scripts for relaxation. (A recording of these scripts by the author is available.) Support groups are described and discussed in Chapter Three. Groups come in many styles and formats—you are urged to find one that feels comfortable to you.

Chapter Four contains the beginning of activities that are helpful for coping. These include journaling or writing in a diary, several structured writing instruments that are designed to organize your thinking, the use of videotaping and autobiographies, art therapy, and rituals and ceremonies. Some of these activities you would do alone, whilst others require organizing with other people.

The heart of this book is Chapter Five where many varieties of coping are discussed, some in much detail. How do you survive in a hospital, cope with insurance companies, communicate with family and friends and medical personnel, set up a support network, and live and die well? In the Alice-in-Wonderland world of a serious disease, many things change in your life. These are not only the physical manifestations of the disease, but also relationships with others and, most importantly, your sense of self. Chapter Five provides guidance in dealing with these matters.

Nutrition is always important. The knowledge and experience of H. Ira Fritz, Ph.D. in this area is a plus. There are many appendices with helpful information including: a sample living will, a sample durable power of attorney for health care, and websites and phone numbers of resources.

Mario Uribe's illustrations provide a pleasant punctuation of the many themes in this book. Mario and I talked about this project over fifteen years ago, and it is wonderful to have him 'illuminate' the text.

Members of the Charlie Brown Exceptional Patient Support Group of Dayton have been helpful in reading some portions of the material, but mainly in their love and support of me as a person. Jane Brown has read the book in its entirety and her comments were helpful. Bernie Siegel supplied a number of useful suggestions. K'Anna Burton's sharing of her surgery story is appreciated. I owe special thanks to my friend Carol E. Dixon. Her comments, based on her experience in helping establish and administer hospice of Dayton, shaped the style and content of this book. Almost every page bears the mark of her suggestions.

Your comments are always welcome. My e-mail address is: rubin.battino@wright.edu.

Rubin Battino
Yellow Springs, Ohio

Foreword

Rubin and I met at a Milton Erickson Congress some years ago. Milton was an American psychiatrist and genius hypnotherapist who translated Freud's great insight about the unconscious determinants of behavior into practical applications that changed people's behaviors. His great talent was in finding a common language of symbols and stories that spoke directly to every patient's unconscious. He helped people understand how to create new endings to old stories by using indirect suggestion, prescribing rituals, even ordeals, and creating sacred objects.

I first visited Milton in the 1970s after working for several years with Native American people. It was in Indian country that I first became exposed to the use of ceremony, myths and symbols in the healing process, and it was Milton who helped me make sense of what I was seeing. Connect with people and you can trigger the mind to abandon old certainties with new possibilities. This is also what Rubin has done in this book.

This is a guide for making connections with people facing serious illness and for those who care for them. It is a practical handbook that uses symbols, ceremonies and science to help people confront their realities and gain new perspectives in dealing with them. It will prepare the mind, body and spirit to face life challenges. This is a book about healing and not curing, about coming to every day as if it has something to teach us.

I encourage you to use the material in this book and customize it in ways that make sense to you. You can share it or send it to friends. It is intended as a gift, and if it works, let Rubin know how you've used it. The bibliography and websites are also useful references that will promote joy on your healing journey.

Carl A. Hammerschlag, M.D.

Contributors

Rubin Battino, M.S.
Rubin has a private practice in Yellow Springs and teaches courses for the Department of Human Services at Wright State University where he holds the rank of adjunct professor. This book is based in part on one of those courses. Rubin has over eight years of experience as a volunteer facilitator in a Bernie Siegel style support group for people who have life-challenging diseases and those who support them, together with many years of experience in individual work with people who have life-challenging diseases. He is President of the Milton H. Erickson Society of Dayton and co-author with T.L. South, Ph.D., of *Ericksonian Approaches: A Comprehensive Manual*, a basic text on Ericksonian hypnotherapy and psychotherapy. Rubin has also written *Guided Imagery and Other Approaches to Healing*. He is Professor Emeritus of Chemistry at Wright State University.

H. Ira Fritz, Ph.D.
Ira received his B.A. in Zoology and his Ph.D. in Nutrition from the University of California at Davis. He was an NIH Postdoctoral Fellow at the University of Pennsylvania. He has taught nutrition at the University of Pennsylvania and at Wright State University. His 35 years of teaching experience have included undergraduate, graduate, nursing, veterinary, and medical students. He is currently Professor Emeritus in the Department of Biochemistry and Molecular Biology at Wright State University. He is also Core Faculty Professor at the Union Institute in Cincinnati, Ohio. Ira authored the chapter on nutrition in *Guided Imagery and Other Approaches to Healing*.

Mario Uribe
Mario Uribe has been drawing and painting since he was three years old. He attended The California Institute of the Arts on a full scholarship, and graduated in 1971. Since then, he has worked as a professional artist with more than 25 years of specializing in the health care field. His paintings, murals, prints, and sculpture help create healing environments in hospitals and clinics from Anchorage, Alaska to San Diego, California. He has won several mural

competitions in California, his native state, and his works form part of both private and public museum collections around the world. He is an ardent lifetime student of traditional Japanese arts like calligraphy, tea ceremony and theater. Mario and his wife Liz travel often to Japan as teachers and guides for The American School of Japanese Arts.

Chapter One
Introduction

1.1 Introduction

Life can be capricious and unpredictable and has a way of challenging us in the most surprising ways. Some of these surprises are pleasant and others are not; some we have some control over after the event. The *Serenity Prayer* counsels, "Grant me the serenity to accept the things I cannot change, the courage to change the things I can, and the wisdom to know the difference." The late Viennese psychiatrist Viktor E. Frankl advised that we always have the choice of *how* we respond to adversity, even in the most extreme of circumstances like his survival of Nazi concentration camps or Christopher Reeve's responses to a riding accident that left him a quadriplegic.

How do you cope with a life-challenging disease or with a catastrophic personal event? Some people seem to be 'naturally' better at this than others, but we can all learn and improve our coping skills. This book is a practical compendium of many ways of coping that I have learned from my friends in the support groups I facilitate, and from my readings and other experiences. This book is for the layperson who is thus challenged, and those who care for them.

How you respond to adversity can have a profound effect on the physical course of a disease. Later in this chapter we cite David Spiegel et al.'s work with fourth-stage metastatic breast cancer women. The field of psychoneuroimmunology (PNI) has unequivocally demonstrated the existence of mind/body interactions. Yet, aside from the scientific evidence, common sense and daily observation provide proof that those who see a glass of water as 'half full' rather than 'half empty' appear to do better in all aspects of life. There is a healing power in hope, and a destructive power in despair. There is healing when you feel in charge and in control, and potential negative effects when you feel hopeless and out of control

1

and dependent. Attitude matters; activity matters; faith and hope matter; people and love and caring and touching and laughter and a baby's smile matter. This moment matters—this moment and this breath and this feeling *are* life. The past is memory and the future is unknown and unexperienced since it is a projection, a dream. Now *is*. And yet, we shouldn't belittle hopes and dreams, for they are the foundation for meaning, and without meaning—life is meaningless, isn't it?

So, this book is about hope—to cope you need hope.

We start with a discussion of the useful distinctions between dis-ease and illness, and between cure and healing.

1.2 Disease/Cure and Illness/Healing

Despite the ancient adage of "sticks and stones can break your bones, but words can never hurt you," words can have powerful positive *and* negative effects on the human mind and body. 'Disease' may mean one thing to one person and something else to another. Oncologists rarely use the word 'cure.' If you have been in remission for five years, then they consider the return of cancer to be unlikely. But they always caution about a possible recurrence. Words and how we interpret them are important, so in this section we define and explore the meanings of four significant words.

It is popular in some quarters to write the word 'disease' as dis-ease, implying that it describes a state that is the opposite of being at ease, in comfort, or relaxed. In this book we define a *disease* as something that is physically wrong with the body. That is, a disease is the pathology itself. Examples are: cancer, infections, hormonal imbalances, diverticulitis, ulcers, strokes, myocardial infarctions and insufficiencies, and broken bones. Reversing or fixing a disease (in Western societies) typically involves a 'mechanical' intervention of some sort: surgery, chemotherapy, radiation, antibiotics, supplements, diet changes, physical rehabilitation, and drugs. When the disease is fixed or has gone away, the person is said to be 'cured.' So, a *cure* is the reversal of a disease, the disappearance of its physical manifestations, and a return to normal healthy functioning. We are fortunate that there are a great many diseases that can be cured in a straightforward manner. We are also fortunate that there are now many ways to ease suffering.

How is healing different from curing? To clarify this, we first need to make a distinction between an illness and a disease. We define *illness* to be the *meaning* that you personally attribute to the disease. These meanings are unique to you and are determined by your history-culture-religion-ethnicity-belief system-intellectual predilection-upbringing-heritage-philosophy of life. Siblings are more likely to interpret a given disease in the same way compared to people from different cultures. Yet, due to different life experiences, sisters may react in very different ways to a preliminary diagnosis of breast cancer. *Healing* applies to the *meaning* of the disease, i.e., the illness. The root of healing signifies 'to make whole.' Healing is more related to internal feeling states than to physical states.

For example, a few decades ago in the Bronx in my Greek-Jewish subculture, the word 'cancer' was rarely mentioned, or spoken only in a whisper. There was a belief that saying the word out loud (or even *thinking* it!) would catch the attention of the 'Evil One' and *you* would then be more susceptible to getting cancer. Evil Ones or devils were part of the belief system of my relatives. This reaction to a word colored all of our thinking and responses. A person who had CANCER was doomed to a horrible death, but it also bore connotations of shame and pity. The *illness* was worse than the disease; it led to a helplessness and hopelessness on the part of the afflicted person, as well as caregivers and well-wishers. Thankfully, many of our attitudes towards 'cancer-the-disease' have changed. Bernie Siegel sums it up best by saying, "Cancer is not a sentence, it is just a word."

Healing deals with attitudes and meaning. When a person is healed, he becomes whole again, and can be at peace with himself, the disease, and the world at large.[1] Healing is involved with the spirit and the soul and one's essence. For some, a healing experience may be described as a spiritual experience, perhaps even a spiritual transformation. To become whole, to be in harmony, to be centered, to find one's true self, to be at peace with yourself and the world—all of these are manifestations of healing.

Figure 1.1a: The word 'cancer' is whispered.

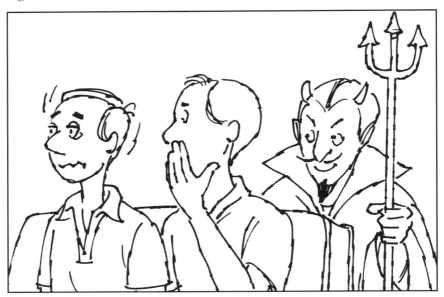

Figure 1.1b: Doctor: "Remember, cancer is just a word—it is not a sentence."

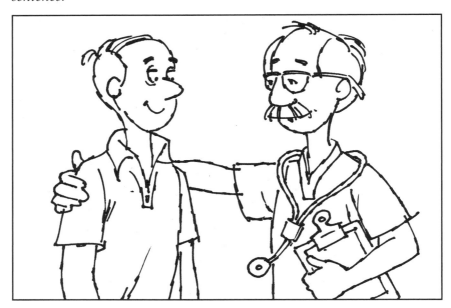

Remarkably, although healing is an end in itself, healing is often accompanied by some degree of curing, if not complete cures, with sufficient frequency to be taken seriously. The goal of healing work is not a cure—the cure is a by-product of healing. In fact, if the sole motivation for healing work is a cure, then the healing work becomes contaminated and side-tracked. Healing invariably involves a search for meaning, a spiritual quest. What does it all mean? Why am I alive at this moment in time? Are there things that are meant for me to do in the rest of my life? About two thousand years ago Rabbi Hillel was asked to summarize his lifelong wisdom. He responded with the following three questions:

> If I am not for myself, who will be?
> If I am only for myself, what am I?
> If not now, when?

We might say that healing an illness involves answering these questions honestly.

A related linguistic pairing are the words 'patient' and 'client.' The linguistic root of patient is in suffering and, in seeking healing, we 'suffer' through to a resolution. In this sense, there is an *active* suffering, rather than a *victim* suffering. Most doctors use the word 'patient' rather than 'client.' Perhaps this is because in so many medical settings a person has to be *patient* in *waiting* for a treatment. The word 'patient' implies a one-down position, superior/inferior, an unequal status. The word 'client' is better since it implies providing a professional service for a fee. *Clients* 'hire' professionals to carry out a specific function such as: write a will, set a bone, fix a leak, and identify and cure an infection. These are contracted services and the professional *works for you*. Which professionals routinely keep you waiting for the service for which you pay them? It is almost as if your time is not as valuable as that of the physician or lawyer or ... Occasional waits for medical services would be reasonable due to unforeseen circumstances. But, waiting seems to be the rule rather than the exception. I had a dentist in Chicago who always had me in the chair at the appointed time. He had an emergency repair at one of these sessions and asked my permission to take care of that client first. He treated his clients with respect, just as I responded to his request with respect. In the patient position, procedures are generally *done to you*. As a client, there would be more cooperation in what happens. In relation to medical practices, it is wise, and even healing, to be a client rather than a patient.

1.3 Complementary and Nontraditional Approaches: Alternative Medicine and Therapies

Bernie Siegel rightly insists that your healing/curing journey needs to be done in *partnership* with traditional medicine. After all, there are a great many diseases that can be competently and effectively treated by modern medicine. These range from fractures to by-pass surgery, (most) infections, hernias, allergies, and cataract surgery. While it is true that the most significant contributor to the increase in longevity since 1900 has been public sanitation, the armamentarium and skills and contributions of present-day physicians are indisputable. One would be foolish indeed not to avail himself of such proven services. Yet, somehow, parallel with the advances of medicine, we find increasing interest in nontraditional approaches to health and health care. Why is this?

Although great progress has been made in many areas, there are still many diseases like the common cold which continue to defy modern medicine. Since hope springs eternal, and you recall your Aunt Mary who had this tonic that always worked in your family, why not try it? There are many folk remedies and traditional Asian herbal medicines that have been used for centuries. There is *occasional* scientific evidence, i.e., double-blind studies, for some of these substances. But, mostly, the evidence for efficaciousness is historical and anecdotal. One advantage of most (but not all) of these substances is that side-effects appear to be minimal. 'Above all, cause no harm to your patients.'

Non-modern-medicine approaches have been called 'complementary,' 'nontraditional,' and 'alternative.' Each of these words has advantages and disadvantages, but since they all convey the sense of being different from standard traditional Western medicine I think they can be used interchangeably—let your preference guide you. Another way to describe these approaches is *transpersonal medicine* (Lawlis, 1997).

Historically, scientific Western medicine is quite young. It can probably be dated from Semmelweis's introduction of antiseptic practices, Pasteur's germ theory of disease, and Morton's use of diethyl ether for anesthesia. This makes modern medicine a little over one century old. Until this time, the medicine that was practiced worldwide was based on historical traditions in each culture. Native Americans have a rich lore of natural products, as well as various healing rites. This is also true in China, Africa, South America, India, and even in Europe. The 19th century apothecaries in London, Vienna, and Philadelphia contained many of the same substances, almost all of them 'natural.' Trial and error was the 'scientific' basis proving the efficacy of these materials.

Before the development of Western medicine, practitioners relied on giving patients many of the same natural or synthetic materials in use today. Their primitive surgical methods were sometimes successful. But the advent of scientific medicine led to an emphasis on 'mechanical' interventions (surgery and drugs) and ignored the mental, spiritual, belief, and meaning sides of both healing and curing. To be sure, physicians had to be aware of exceptional patients who got well without their help. A scientist understands cause and effect: splinting a broken bone leads to its proper knitting together; a by-pass operation improves heart capacity; an antibiotic rids the body of an infection. But where does an AIDS or cancer patient who becomes symptom free without medical care fit in? How do you explain Norman Cousins' cure from ankylosing spondilitis? How can sand paintings and psychosurgery help? By what mechanisms do acupuncture and hypnosis let patients undergo major operations pain free?

Western medicine has separated the mind from the body. The much older, traditional medical practices made no such distinctions— man was a whole: integrated mind *and* body *and* spirit. Viktor Frankl (1959, 1962) repeatedly stated in his lectures that physicians treat only the body, psychologists and psychiatrists the mind, and that both ignore the third dimension of the spirit or soul. In Frankl's sense, you can't really be a *healer* if you deal with only one aspect of the mind/body/spirit continuum. They are inseparable. There may be times when, for convenience, you deal with just one part, but that is done for whose convenience? Native healers, shamans and witch doctors have always dealt with the whole person—how can you be in *harmony* with yourself and nature as isolated parts?

Organized and personal religions have used prayer as a method to attain healing and cures. To simplify, prayer has been basically used in four ways. The *first* is simply a way of a person talking to God or a supreme being or spirit: a way to communicate with something or someone beyond themselves—a sharing of their inner thoughts with this external presence. The *second* is to ask this external and knowledgeable and powerful entity for help in a specific concern. These concerns range from mundane specific items (winning the lottery, passing an exam, appropriate weather) to the correction of physical ailments to attain cures. In some way, the justice of your cause or plea is recognized and the all-powerful all-knowing being or entity directly intercedes on your behalf. When someone has a life-challenging disease, this second type of prayer appears to be the most common. The *third* form of prayer is more spiritual, and is a kind of meditation whose result is some degree of fusion with, or knowledge of, the universal spirit. A *fourth* form of prayer is the simple 'thank you' that is part of saying grace or just a way of showing appreciation. Belief systems can have powerful influences on our lives. (See Dossey (1993) for more information on prayer.)

The search for meaning drives many people. When a person functions with that meaning directing his life, there can be profound physical and psychological effects. This quest has been expressed in different ways: (1) Viktor Frankl as a search for meaning; (2) Joseph Campbell as finding and following your bliss; and (3) Lawrence LeShan as discovering and singing your own unique song. The quest involves identifying your hopes, dreams, and unfulfilled desires. What is it that you've always wanted to do or be? Bernie Siegel tells the story of a lawyer who had 'terminal' cancer. This man became a lawyer to please his father. Faced with a limited life, he gave up his law practice and returned to his first love of playing the violin. The cancer disappeared and he found a new career as a professional musician. Will this always be the case? Of course not. Yet, at the minimum, finding and singing your own unique song can lead to healing. Why wait for a diagnosis of something like cancer to send you on your quest?

The lawyer's story is 'anecdotal evidence' of the power of the mind, the spirit. As such, it is inadmissible in the court of modern medicine. Yet every physician could tell you such stories about his own patients, i.e., people who underwent, for no scientifically known reason, complete remission or cures. The National Center for Complementary and Alternative Medicine (NCCAM) of the National Institutes of Health (NIH) is currently funding such research activities. The study of exceptions has led to many discoveries.

Lawrence LeShan (1989) in the introductory chapter to *Cancer as a Turning Point* cites many sources prior to 1900 that connect cancer to hopelessness and deep anxiety and disappointment. Although hopelessness is certainly a factor in cancer, *it is only one factor*. Knowledge of this was the basis for LeShan's approach to working with people who have cancer, to have them find and sing their own 'unique song.' Bernie Siegel has frequently stated, "What's wrong with hope?" (Appendix A lists LeShan's 31 significant questions (1989, pp. 161–165) as a guide to your personal work.)

An excellent book on alternative treatment for cancer is the one by Lerner (1996). This book is based to a large extent on a governmental study (U.S. Congress Office of Technology Assessment, Unconventional Cancer Therapies, 1990). *All* of the alternative treatments that Lerner writes about have in fact helped *some* people. The outcomes are neither consistent nor predictable because people are unique. Pharmacopeias can give you the dose for the *average* person of a given body weight, but, this will be an overdose for some people and ineffectively low for others. For those with cancer, Lerner's book does give balanced and well-researched guidelines to alternative/complementary treatments.

The psychiatrist David Spiegel (1989, et seq.) has now provided definitive proof that a psychotherapeutic support group is effective for last-stage breast cancer. The women in the support group lived about twice as long beyond the start of the study as the women in the control group. It is not clear why the support group had this effect, although the original study has been replicated. The next section is devoted to a summary of it. There may be more detail here than you need, but the work is so important that it needs to be accurately described. You may even wish to show a copy of this section to your physician.

1.4 *David Spiegel's Research*

The title of Spiegel et al.'s landmark paper (1989) is *Effect of psychosocial treatment on survival of patients with metastatic breast cancer.* In the introduction they state:

> Our objective was to assess whether group therapy in patients with metastatic breast cancer had any effect on survival.... We started with the belief that positive psychological and symptomatic effects could occur without affecting the course of the disease: we expected to improve the quality of life without affecting its quantity.

Their surprising results can be ascertained from the *summary* in their article. (N = number of people; SD = standard deviation.)

> The effect of psychosocial intervention of survival on 86 patients with metastatic breast cancer was studied prospectively. The 1 year intervention consisted of weekly supportive group therapy with self-hypnosis for pain. Both the treatment (N = 50) and control groups (N = 36) had routine oncological care. At 10 year follow-up, only 3 of the patients were alive, and death records were obtained for the other 83. Survival from time of randomization and onset of intervention was a mean 36.6 (SD 37.6) months in the intervention group compared with 18.9 (SD 10.8) months in the control group, a significant difference. Survival plots indicated that divergence in survival began at 20 months after entry, or 8 months after intervention ended.

Another way of examining their results is to reproduce their Table III (Spiegel et al. 1989) on survival in months with given Mean (SD):

	Control	**Intervention**
Survival from:		
Study entry to death	18.9 (10.8)	36.6 (37.6)
Initial medical visit to death	81.2 (53.9)	94.6 (61.0)
First metastasis to death	43.2 (20.5)	85.4 (45.4)

Each of these categories is interesting in its own way. Perhaps the middle entry is most significant, indicating an almost seven year period from the initial medical visit to death for everyone in the control group, and that members of the intervention group survived 13 months longer on average. Most surprising may be the fact that three members of the intervention group were alive at the

10-year follow-up. Despite criticism of the research (1989, Letters to the Editor, two citations), the research was solidly based and was the first real evidence of the effectiveness of psychosocial interventions. (This work has since been replicated by Spiegel and co-workers and others.)

Figure 1.2: Psychotherapy support groups work.

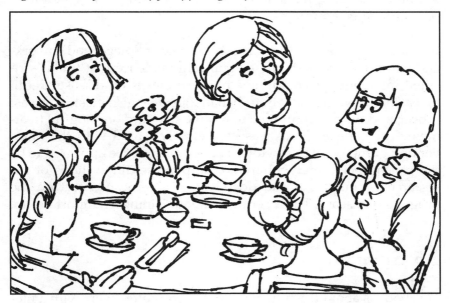

It is also worth quoting here in its entirety the nature of the intervention:

> The intervention lasted for a whole year while both control and treatment groups received their routine oncological care. The three intervention groups met weekly for 90 minutes, led by a psychiatrist or social worker with a therapist who had breast cancer in remission. The groups were structured to encourage discussion of how to cope with cancer, but at no time were patients led to believe that participation would affect the course of disease. Group therapy patients were encouraged to come regularly and express their feelings about the illness and its effect on their lives. Physical problems, including side-effects of chemotherapy or radiotherapy, were discussed and a self-hypnosis strategy was taught for pain control (Spiegel, 1985). Social isolation was countered by developing strong relations among members. Members encouraged one another to be

more assertive with doctors. Patients focused on how to extract meaning from tragedy by using their experience to help other patients and their families. One major function of the leaders was to keep the group directed toward facing the grieving losses.

The emphasis of this program was on "living as fully as possible, improving communication with family members and doctors, facing and mastering fears about death and dying, and controlling pain and other symptoms."

It is hard to overemphasize the significance of Spiegel and cowork-ers' work. Here was the first significant evidence that 'mind'-oriented interventions could have physical effects on disease. Recall that *all* of the women in the study had fourth-stage metastatic breast cancer, and they all continued to receive standard oncological treatment. The control group was very closely paired with the intervention group on many factors. The only difference appeared to be the psychosocial intervention. So, despite the initial thesis of the researchers, mind can and does have a significant effect on the progress of disease. Think seriously about joining a support group.

1.5 Summary

This book is about teaching you how to cope effectively with a life-challenging disease. Many practical examples will be given later. This introduction emphasizes the power of hope and words and psychotherapeutic support. The mind and what you think can have a positive effect on outcomes.

Note

[1] Generally, masculine pronouns will be used in odd-numbered chapters, and feminine pronouns in the even-numbered ones.

Chapter Two
Relaxation Methods

2.1 *Introduction*

Relaxation can enhance the immune system. The so-called 'relaxation response' hit public awareness with Benson's landmark book (1975) on the subject. Here was a simple, noninvasive meditative technique that (according to the jacket blurb): "… will unlock your hidden assets and help you: relieve inner tensions; deal more effectively with stress; lower blood pressure; (and) improve your physical and emotional health." These may appear on the surface to be the assertions of a snake-oil salesman, but Benson cited careful studies demonstrating that these effects are indeed real for the relaxation response. In addition to the above, relaxation also: enhances immune system function, lowers oxygen consumption and the respiratory rate, decreases the heart rate and blood pressure (in those with elevated blood pressure), increases alpha waves, and decreases muscle tension. Relaxation really is beneficial in a variety of ways.

There are many ways to attain a relaxed state. Among the more common are: Transcendental Meditation, Zen practices and yoga, autogenic training, progressive relaxation, and hypnosis. It apparently makes little difference in the final analysis which technique you use. My preferred approach (including a transcript) is given at the end of the chapter. Also, at the end of the chapter are three guided imagery healing meditations.

Transcendental Meditation is a school of meditation involving classes and trainers and an individual mantra (special word or phrase) for repetition. *Zen* meditation is a discipline taught by a Zen master and involves much repetitive practice. One part of training in *yoga* involves the physical positions, and another part involves a meditative practice. *Autogenic Training* (Linden, 1990) is based on learning six mental exercises for daily practice until they become almost automatic. *Hypnosis* and *self-hypnosis* with suggestions for deep relaxation also work well. A common denominator in all approaches is that you get better at meditating with practice, i.e., you can attain deeper states more quickly.

2.2 Jacobson's Progressive Relaxation

The Jacobson progressive relaxation method was devised by a University of Chicago physician/physiologist in the 1930s (Jacobson, 1938). The name is descriptive of the process. Typically starting with the feet, you say to yourself (or follow a guide), "Now tense the muscles in your left foot. Then relax them. Now tense the muscles in your right foot. Then relax them (or release the tension)." You then progress, alternating up your legs to the abdomen, the buttocks, the back, the chest, hands and arms and shoulders, to the neck, and the head. Practitioners differ on the number of muscle groups. The tension is typically held for a few seconds before releasing. A passive attitude while lying down in a quiet room is helpful. The process may end with tensing the entire body before releasing, perhaps with a deep sigh. Progressive relaxation teaches you to recognize through tension-and-release how to be able to release muscular tensions arising in any part of the body. The procedure is widely used.

You will notice in Section 2.5 where I present my recommended method for relaxing, that I make no use of the progressive relaxation approach. A better way to do progressive relaxation would be to first experience the sensations of tension and relaxation with *one* group of muscles on both sides of the body—making a fist would be a good starting point. Then, starting with the feet just let all the muscles there relax, become soft and comfortable and at ease. Then continue emphasizing comfort and ease and softness and lightness, for all of the other muscle groups in your body, ending with a total body sense of calm and relaxation (perhaps, with an audible sigh).

2.3 Benson's Relaxation Response Method

Benson (1975) found that there were four common components for eliciting the relaxation. The *first* is a quiet environment, i.e., the phone is disconnected, people are told not to disturb you, and you use a backroom away from street noise. The *second* is an object to dwell upon. This may be: repeating a sound or word, gazing fixedly at an object, or concentrating upon a particular feeling or sensation. Since there will *always* be distracting thoughts, you return to your focus over and over again. (With practice, fewer distracting thoughts emerge.) The *third* component is a passive attitude. Benson considers a passive attitude to be the most important component. The quiet environment and object of focus aid in this, as does the *fourth* element of a comfortable position. The recommended position is sitting, since lying down may lead to sleep, which is okay in itself, but not the goal of learning to attain and use the relaxation response. The process is not complicated, although a teacher can be helpful.

In Benson's 1996 book he devotes an entire chapter (pp. 123–148) to the relaxation response. His Table 2 (p. 131) gives a comparison between the fight-or-flight response and the relaxation response. It is summarized below.

Physiologic State	Fight-or-Flight Response	Relaxation Response
Metabolism	increases	decreases
Blood pressure	increases	decreases
Heart rate	increases	decreases
Rate of breathing	increases	decreases
Blood flowing to the muscles of the arms and legs	increases	stable
Muscle tension	increases	decreases
Slow brain waves	decreases	increases

Benson states that there are only two basic steps to elicit the relaxation response: (1) repeat a word, sound, prayer, phrase, or muscular activity; and (2) passively disregard everyday thoughts that come to mind, and return to your repetition. He states that their research has found that performing a focused exercise activates the relaxation response. Benson teaches the following nine-step generic technique (p. 136) to his patients.

Step 1. Pick a focus word or short phrase that's firmly rooted in your belief system.
Step 2. Sit quietly in a comfortable position.

Step 3.   Close your eyes.

Step 4.   Relax your muscles.

Step 5.   Breathe slowly and naturally, and as you do, repeat your focus word, phrase, or prayer silently to yourself as you exhale.

Step 6.   Assume a passive attitude. Don't worry about how well you're doing. When other thoughts come to mind, simply say to yourself, "Oh, well," and gently return to the repetition.

Step 7.   Continue for 10 to 20 minutes.

Step 8.   Do not stand immediately. Continue sitting quietly for a minute or so, allowing other thoughts to return. Then open your eyes and sit for another minute before rising.

Step 9.   Practice this technique once or twice daily.

The above is a good and well-founded basic approach to relaxation.

2.4 *Meditation*

Meditations have been part of all religions in some way through all times. Our image of holy persons involves seeing them at their meditations. You can learn how to meditate by studying Lawrence LeShan's book (1974), particularly Chapter Eight on *The 'How' of Meditation.* This excellent book comes with an audiotape and guide. The meditation of breath counting is the simplest one. LeShan recommends, "you strive to be aware of just your counting and to be as fully aware of it as possible." He also recommends counting the exhalations, and then repeating. If you count both inhalation and exhalation, you can add an 'and' between each number. Pick a number to count up to and a duration before you start. You can begin with 15 minutes of daily practice and slowly move up to 30 minutes. LeShan also discusses other styles of meditation. Meditation is an excellent way to elicit the relaxation response.

2.5 *How to Relax*

In this section you will be given some detailed directions on how to relax, including a relaxation script. The popular notion of relaxing

Figure 2.1: Relaxing.

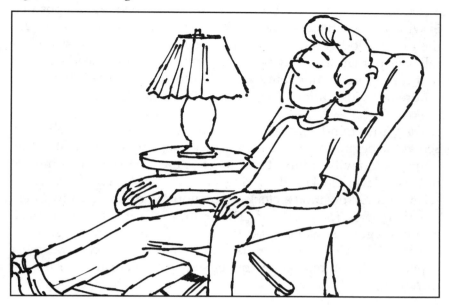

is coming home from work, kicking off your shoes, getting into comfortable clothes, having a drink, and 'relaxing' in a comfortable chair with the paper or watching television. This undoubtedly involves getting into an easier, quieter and calmer state of mind, but it is not what we have in mind as relaxation, which is a more structured and conscious activity. The parts of the relaxation process follow:

a. *Quiet Space.* It is important to be undisturbed for the 15 minutes or so you need. A room without a phone or with it unplugged is a beginning. (Remember that just unhooking a phone frequently results in that endless beeping signal.) Other people in the house/apartment need to be told about your quiet time and that you are not to be disturbed. A room away from street noise is helpful, particularly if you need to leave the window open. Soft lighting is better than bright lights; some people prefer the dark—you must suit yourself in this regard. When you are experienced at relaxing, you can do this in almost any environment as long as you are not directly disturbed—the environment becomes a kind of 'white' noise.

b. *Comfortable Position.* Generally, a sitting posture with a straight back is best. This prevents falling asleep and promotes easy breathing. Really flexible people may adopt the lotus posture using a cushion or a low stool. Use any chair, couch, bed, or any position in which you will feel comfortable and without any body strain for the time period you have chosen. If you are so relaxed that you do fall asleep, then that may be what your mind/body needs most at that time. You are not being graded on how you relax. There is no failure here, just different ways to attain the same goal.

c. *Time*. Your mind contains a remarkably accurate clock. Tell yourself at the beginning of the session just how long you wish it to last. Your session will end itself within a minute or two of that time. Do not use alarm clocks—their ring or buzz can be startling. If you wish, you can position a clock where you can easily see it by opening your eyes for a second. The optimum duration for a relaxation/imagery session appears to be about 15 minutes. As a beginner, 10 to 15 minutes is sufficient. As you become more experienced, you may enjoy longer sessions. There are no rules for duration.

d. *Eyes Open or Closed*. Most people do best to close their eyes during a session because that greatly reduces the amount of sensory input. If you are uncomfortable with closed eyes, then staring at an object and/or defocusing your eyes are just as effective in limiting input. You may even experience 'tunnel vision' with defocused eyes. Again, there are no rules—do what is comfortable and normal for you.

e. *Object of Focus*. The relaxation process works most smoothly when there is something to focus your mind on, to contemplate, if you will. This can be a physical object such as a spot on the wall, a candle, a picture or part of a picture, or a flower. You may focus on a particular sound you make like: 'Om,' a mantra, or a phrase that is repeated like 'God is good,' or 'God is One,' or 'Peace,' or a nonsense phrase like lah-dee. Simply focus on counting breaths. Although LeShan recommends a count of four, you may count to any number you wish before returning to one. To avoid monotony vary the count. You may count the inbreath and the outbreath or both. This is a matter of personal preference. When counting breaths try focusing on the end of your nose, sensing the cooler inbreath and the warmer and moister outbreath—this extra point of concentration limits potentially distracting sensory input.

As you become more experienced, there are fewer distracting thoughts. But, there are *always* such random thoughts drifting through your mind. Simply acknowledge the presence of the thought, thank it, and go back to 'one'. Some days there will be many such temptations to distract you—thank the thought *and* go back to 'one'. If the thoughts become too insistent, this means that this was not a good time for a meditative session, so just stop it. Such an experience is just another way to learn about yourself. *Forcing* yourself to relax is like forcing yourself to be spontaneous ...

f. *Imagery Work.* You have now paid attention to the 'mechanical' factors involved in relaxing. By whatever method you pick, after seven to 10 minutes of relaxation you are ready to start on your imagery work if you so choose (imagery work is optional). Without looking at a clock, you either program your internal clock to let you know it is time to begin or, better, you just know by your physical quietude and the ease and softness of your breathing and a period with no distracting thoughts, that this is imagery time. This inner knowledge of when to start comes with practice—you will find an unique sense of it for yourself.

The imagery work itself incorporates the specific visualizations, words, or sensations that you have an inner sense are appropriate and helpful for you. This imagery may be developed by you, with a guide, or adapted from the many ritual images presented in Achterberg et al. (1994), Naparstek (1994), or from some other source. In particular, Naparstek (Image Paths, 24200 Chagrin Boulevard, Suite 240, Beachwood, OH 44122; 800-800-8661) has produced a variety of quality guided imagery tapes. Generally, the more vivid and detailed the image, the better it works. That is, it is important for you to be engrossed in your own imagery. For some people, observing the image working in your body from a dissoci-ated perspective is the mode of choice. Also, for some, generalized directions like "Okay, immune system, just get in there and do what it takes to get rid of this disease" are the preferred approach. Again, the imagery work is unique to the individual.

The imagery portion of the session lasts from seven to 12 minutes, ending at a natural place for you. For more information on guided imagery, see Battino (2000).

g. *Reorientation*. Loud noises or interruptions while you are in a relaxed state can activate the startle reflex. Reorient yourself slowly to the waking state. You can give yourself suggestions about ending the session with a few deep breaths, blinking your eyes, stretching, and returning to the present with an inner calm.

2.6 *Relaxation Script*

Hello! This is a tape designed to help you relax into a comfortable and calm state. Please be sure you are sitting or reclining in a way that is easy for you, and that you are in a quiet place, with nothing to bother you and nothing to disturb you. This is your quiet time, a peaceful one, a special time just for you. If at any time you need to move or adjust your position to be even more comfortable, please do so. I may not be using just the right words for you now, or saying them in just the right way—please feel free to change the words and how you hear them, so that they are just the best for you at this time …

And you can continue your relaxation by paying attention to your breathing, noticing each breath in, and each breath out. Slowly and easily, calmly, just breathing in a soft natural way. In and out. Notice how the cooler air enters and warmer moister air leaves. Simply, softly, breathing. Perhaps counting your breaths—one … and … two … and … three … and … four … and … five … and, back to one … two … three …

If any stray thoughts should wander through your mind, notice them, observe them, thank them, and then go back to … one … and … two … and … three … That's right. Safely moving and drifting with each easy calming breath. Softly. Simply. Naturally. Your time. Your safe secure quiet time. Breathing easily. Enjoying this moment, now. This breath, this peaceful time and place. Softly breathing. Such calm, such peace. This breath … and the next one … your time … your quiet time … a healing space and place … allowing this peace to fill you. Your peaceful time. Relaxing even more. Yes. Another easy breath. And another. Enjoying.

And within your mind now, you can just drift off to some safe and secure place, one that is uniquely yours. It may be real, or just real within your imagination ... your place ... a special place ... peaceful and calm ... serene ... There may be music ... your music ... You may be alone or with someone special ... or with many ... your time ... your place ... safe and secure and serene ... relaxing even more ... You become so engrossed that time almost stops ... enjoying just being ... your place ... peace ... And you can return here whenever you wish ... remembering ... taking time for yourself ... a few quiet breaths ... relaxing ... drifting off ... safely ...

[Pause] And, when you are ready, find yourself taking a deep breath or two, stretching, and blinking your eyes. And you can come back now, to this room, feeling ever so relaxed, so at ease, rested. Yes. Thank you.

The previous example may be spoken to you by someone you know, or you may wish to make a tape of it for yourself. Your quiet time. Thank you. (The single ellipsis indicates a short pause, and more ellipses indicate longer pauses.)

Three general healing imagery scripts follow in the next three sections. Again, you can tape them for yourself or have someone read them to you, or purchase the tape accompanying this book.

2.7 *Healing Presence Imagery Script*

Hello. Find a way of being comfortable ... just shift around some now ... moving your head or arms or ... so that you are even more comfortable. Feel free to move at any time ... This is your time, nothing at all to bother you, nothing else to do. Your special quiet time.... And you can begin with paying attention to your breathing ... noticing each breath as it comes in, slightly cooler ... and each exhale ... slightly warmer and moister. Just one breath at a time. Simply, easily. And you may count your breaths. One ... two ... three... four ... five ... And back to one ... two ... three... simply and easily. One breath at a time. Softly. Simply relaxing into that quiet rhythm ... one ... two... three ...

From time to time a stray thought may wander through ... notice it ... thank it ... and go back to ... one ... and two ... and three ... and ... Another thought may come through ... notice it ... and ... yes ...

Thank you ... back to ... Easily and simply, so restful, as you continue to become even more relaxed ... more at ease ... easily ...

And within your mind now, you can drift off to your own special, safe and secure place. I don't know where it is ... or what it is like ... or even if it is real or imaginary ... Just your special ... safe ... healing ... place. A place that is just yours ... Enjoy being there ... noticing, looking around, sensing, hearing ... maybe there are some special odors. Your place ... resting even more fully ...

While you are there, you notice that someone, a special healer, a powerful and knowledgeable healer, is there with you too. Just the two of you.... Sensing that healing presence ... perhaps there is some music or singing or words that are ever so full of meaning.... And I don't know who your special healer is ... this healing presence ... someone from your past, or future, a religious figure ... your healer ... here ... with you.... Just being there, and enjoying being cared for ... your time ... your place ... now ...

And the healer comes close enough to touch you ... gentle, warm, energetic, knowing hands ... and they lightly touch those parts of your body that are in need. And with each touch you can sense, you really feel, a special tingling or warmth, or perhaps coolness, find its way to those places where healing is needed ... eliminating unwanted cells swiftly, easily, automatically ... just as fast as your body can handle this now ... Maybe crushing or destroying or simply eliminating those cells and masses ... the power of the healing presence moving to wherever it is needed, knowing just where to do its work ... yes ... and yes ... and yes ...

And, in those other places where a repairing or rebuilding or reconstructing or rewiring kind of healing is needed, you can sense this healing presence, your healer ... repairing, rebuilding, making appropriate connections and adjustments, simply and easily.... Knowing just where to work, effectively and efficiently ... repairing ... like new ... maybe better ...

Your healer is also a teacher ... improving your immune system ... showing it new and better ways ... reminding of older ways that are still helpful ... teaching ... so that this healing work can go on and on and on ... just as long as you need it.... Remembering ...

learning ... storing away ... Your healer gently completes the work for now ... slowly withdrawing ... a last touch or two ... while you know somewhere deep inside just how this work will continue and continue and continue ... your time ... your healer ...

Thank you for letting me spend this time with you.... When you are ready, you may take a deep breath or two, blink your eyes, stretch, and return to this room ... here and now.

Yes ... Yes ... Yes ...

Figure 2.2: Healing hands imagery.

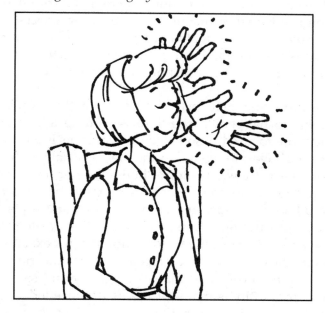

2.8 Healing Light Imagery Script

Hello. Find a way of being comfortable ... just shift around some now ... moving your head or arms or ... so that you are even more comfortable. Feel free to move at any time ... This is your time, nothing at all to bother you, nothing else to do. Your special quiet time.... And you can begin with paying attention to your breathing ... noticing each breath as it comes in, slightly cooler ... and each exhale ... slightly warmer and moister. Just one breath at a time.

Simply, easily. And you may be counting your breaths. One ... two ... three... four ... five ... And back to one ... two ... three... simply and easily. One breath at a time. Softly. Simply relaxing into that quiet rhythm ... one ... two... three ...

From time to time a stray thought may wander through ... notice it ... thank it ... and go back to ... one ... and two ... and three ... and ... Another thought may come through ... notice it ... and ... yes ... Thank you ... back to ... Easily and simply, so restful, as you continue to become even more relaxed ... more at ease ... easily ...

And within your mind now, you can drift off to your own special, safe and secure place. I don't know where it is ... or what it is like ... or even if it is real or imaginary ... just your special ... safe ... healing ... place. A place that is just yours ... Enjoy being there ... noticing, looking around, sensing, hearing ... maybe there are some special odors. Your place ... resting even more fully ...

And enjoy just being there, peacefully and quietly.... An interesting thing begins to happen ... the light is shifting and changing ... becoming more focused in some gentle way. This is a healing light, coming from above and around, somehow, especially for you ... and I don't know exactly what color or hue it is ... or how bright ... or how focused or diffuse the ray or rays ... or just how warm or cool it is ... You know ... and you can adjust it so that it is just right for you now ... just the right intensity.... And this healing light, perhaps from above, has its own way of knowing just exactly where to focus its energies to heal and correct and adjust and rid your body of those unwanted cells and masses ... gently and safely moving through your skin in as many places as it is needed ... and only doing its healing and eliminating work on just those spots and places ... oh, so very carefully and safely selective ... where it is needed ... so easily and gently and softly ... touching, covering, shining, and cleansing your body with rays of hope and energy and power ... your healing light ... and doing this just as fast as your body can get rid of the debris, the fragments, the shriveled and vanishing unwanted cells ... It is almost as if a Higher Power or some Cosmic or Universal Force, something outside you, is beaming on you with love and compassion and healing energy ... working ever so quickly and efficiently ... cleansing, restoring ... yes, restoring, for this healing light with its special colors is restoring and rebuilding … and bathing your healthy cells with extra energy so that they become healthier, and the healthy cells increase naturally and simply … you can almost feel that now, can you not? … how this light is re-energizing your immune system, giving it a boost and renewed vigor, to be alertly protective …. yes, that's right, isn't it? … becoming stronger, doing more, doing more so easily … feeling the healing light all over and through you … your healing …

And when it has done its work for now, the light gently withdraws and fades, leaving you feeling ever so rested and relaxed, yet strangely, full of energy too…. When you are ready you can take a few energizing deep breaths, blink your eyes, open them, and return to this room.

Thank you for letting me spend this time with you…. Yes … Yes …

2.9 *Healing Hands Imagery Script*

Hello. Find a way of being comfortable … just shift around some now … moving your head or arms or … so that you are even more comfortable. Feel free to move at any time … This is your time, nothing at all to bother you, nothing else to do. Your special quiet time…. And you can begin with paying attention to your breathing … noticing each breath as it comes in, slightly cooler … and each exhale … slightly warmer and moister. Just one breath at a time. Simply, easily. And you may be counting your breaths. One … two … three… four … five … And back to one … two … three… simply and easily. One breath at a time. Softly. Simply relaxing into that quiet rhythm … one … two… three …

From time to time a stray thought may wander through … notice it … thank it … and go back to … one … and two … and three … and … Another thought may come through … notice it … and … yes … Thank you … back to … Easily and simply, so restful, as you continue to become even more relaxed … more at ease … easily …

And, within your mind, now, you can drift off to your own special, safe and secure place. I don't know where it is … or what it is like … or even if it is real or imaginary … Just your special … safe … healing … place. A place that is just yours … Enjoy being there …

25

noticing, looking around, sensing, hearing … maybe there are some special odors. Your place … resting even more fully …

Your special place, somewhere, somewhen, with interesting things … enjoying a calm and relaxed time, your time … and, you know, you know just how important touch and being touched is for healing, do you not? … Connections with another, or many others, sensing their caring and love and compassion … and the desire to heal, to help heal, to help your healing in any way possible … And while you rest in your special place, can you not sense now the presence of a pair of healing hands? … slowly coming closer … and I don't know whose hands they are … maybe someone from your past or childhood, maybe a spiritual healer, perhaps the hands of a saint or religious entity … important, powerful, knowledgeable, healing hands … soft and gentle … yet stronger, much stronger than whatever within you needs healing …

And, those hands gently move over your whole body, just an inch or so away, sensing where their healing touch, their healing energy is needed … Then, ever so gently, the hands touch you just in those places where their power is needed … sending healing feelings and energy through your skin to surround and encompass and eliminate those cells and groups of cells … to reduce them … crumble them … so your body can easily get rid of the debris … many places … wherever that healing touch is needed … reaching into all parts of your body … simply, naturally, powerfully … cleansing and clearing and eliminating … just as fast as your body can handle this clean-up work … knowing that this cleansing, healing process will continue … just as long as you need it to … to be healthy and whole again … The magic, the power, of healing hands … yours at this moment … and later … you can still feel that touch working … tonight … tomorrow … next week … and all the way into your future … for you know you can never touch without being touched … the contact brings a kind of fusion of minds and bodies and spirits … sharing, working together, being the more powerful for that touch, that touching experience …

And your body will remember the touch, the touching, of your healing hands … continuing the work long after they've gone to help someone else. And you can sense that the hands do a final gentle scan of your body for now, and then leave …

When you are ready, find yourself waking, returning to this room, full of energy, yet as refreshed as awaking from a satisfying nap. Thank you ... Yes ... Yes ...

2.10 Summary

This chapter has covered some basic relaxation methods and provided a general relaxation script, as well as three general guided imagery healing scripts.

Chapter Three
Support Groups

3.1 *Introduction*

Everyone's needs are different. The group must *feel right* to you on some personal level before you make any commitments about attendance. Most hospitals offer support groups and/or services to people who have cancer or other serious diseases. These hospital-based groups may be solely for the patient, solely for those who support the patient, or for both. These groups are generally free of charge.

There are many support groups organized around a particular disease like emphysema, cancer, colorectal cancer, asthma, etc. These groups are generally associated with a national organization, e.g., The American Cancer Society. Usually there are no fees. Typically, the specialized support group meetings are heavily oriented towards information about the disease and coping with it. Support groups may be classified by the amount of time spent on information and lectures versus the amount of time spent on emotional or psychological support. This is why it is so important to check out support groups, and be open to going to groups with different styles as your own needs change. Above all, it is important to recognize that seeking help and support is an indicator of *strength* on your part, and is one area under your control. Although the members of a particular group may be quite ill indeed, the atmosphere is generally that of hope and courage—they are brave people who have gone through or are going through whatever is your specific disease. You learn from each other's experience. These are generally not 'downer' groups, and there is a surprising amount of humor present—this 'in' group can share jokes or so-called 'black' humor which they would find to be uncomfortable in the presence of healthy people. This is an important point, since a person with a disease frequently feels isolated and different and even stigmatized with respect to 'healthy' people. There is a sense of unreality, of separateness, of estrangement. On some core level they do not recognize themselves—the disease has transformed them into a different and strange person. It is not so long ago that these people were ostracized, isolated, and driven out of their communities. Recall the history of the way that people with leprosy and tuberculosis were treated. Echoes of these old behaviors and fears still reverberate.

There are a number of psychotherapists and social workers and other helping professionals who offer fee-for-service assistance for people who have life-challenging diseases and those who support them. Sometimes this is 'straight' psychotherapy for the individual or their family. Sometimes they offer programs for grieving, and sometimes there are privately run support groups. These groups may reflect the particular orientation of the provider in terms of affiliation, nutrition, body work, and alternatives to conventional medicine. Always remember that you are in control and that the choice to use or stay with a particular practitioner is yours. Michael Lerner's book (1996) is the essential guide to evaluating comple-mentary practices for cancer. As far as I know, there is nothing like Lerner's guide for other diseases.

In this chapter, several specific support groups or styles will be described.

3.2 *David Spiegel's Breast Cancer Support Groups*

Spiegel et al.'s support group (1989) for women with metastatic breast cancer is a classic psychotherapy-based group. (Spiegel et al.'s research is described in Section 1.4.) Such a psychotherapy group is run by a trained psychiatrist, psychologist, counselor, or social worker with typically two leaders working with a group of 10 to 12 participants. Meetings are weekly or biweekly and run for a fixed time period of 10 or 12 sessions, or from three to 12 months. Participants make a commitment to attend all of the sessions. Once a group has started, new members are rarely admitted, since the group quickly establishes an identity and a strong group loyalty. In a disease-based group (versus a psychotherapy-based group), the members are encouraged to be in contact with each other outside of the meetings.

The Spiegel groups met for 90 minutes. Although other groups may meet for longer times, up to three hours per session, it is rare that a group would meet for less than 90 minutes. One reality constraint is that 90 minutes may be as long as a person with an active disease can comfortably attend a meeting. In the Spiegel groups, an extra measure of rapport was attained by having one of the leaders be a person who had breast cancer in remission.

The following quote from the 1989 paper describes the nature of Spiegel et al.'s group interventions:

> The groups were structured to encourage discussion of how to cope with cancer, but at no time were patients led to believe that partici-pation would affect the course of the disease. Group therapy patients were encouraged to come regularly and express their feel-ings about the illness and its effects on their lives. Physical problems ,including side-effects of chemotherapy or radiotherapy, were dis-cussed and a self-hypnosis strategy, was taught for pain control (Spiegel, 1985). Social isolation was countered by developing strong relations among members. Members encouraged one another to be more assertive with doctors. Patients focused on how to extract meaning from tragedy by using their experience to help other patients and their families. One major function of the leaders was to keep the group directed toward facing the grieving losses.

This is a succinct statement of the way these groups functioned. As pointed out in Section 1.4, the results were remarkable—which establishes the effectiveness of psychotherapy-based support groups for working with cancer patients. The Spiegel support groups were run by trained psychotherapists. Although it is not necessary, the inclusion of group leaders who were models of heal-ing, in that they were in remission from the same disease, must have been an important contributory factor.

3.3 Exceptional Cancer Patient (ECaP) Groups

ECaP was started by Bernie Siegel in 1978. His initial motivation came from a patient who said, "I need to know how to live between office visits." Initially, ECaP was financed by Bernie (who prefers to be called by his first name). He later turned it over to others to run, because the demands of his practice and ECaP at the same time became too much, and he wanted ECaP to go on without him. The difficulties that led to changes in ECaP and its movement to its present location (Exceptional Cancer Patients, 522 Jackson Park Drive, Meadville, PA 16355; (814) 337–8192; www.ecap-online.org) started after he left the organization. Dr. Barry Bittman currently oversees the program, which puts out an excellent catalog of materials featuring Bernie's tapes (audio and video) and books. This catalog also offers a fairly comprehensive set of materials of other contributors to the field of alternative and complementary medicine. ECaP puts out a yearly directory of support groups in the U.S.A. that lists individual practitioners and groups, with information on the services provided.

Bernie found that his concern and empathy and hope sustained his patients during their office visits, and he reasoned that regular support group meetings would be of help. The style of the groups evolved. Bernie reports that it took him about six months to learn how to shut up in the groups and *listen* to the members talk. He found that the most important aspect of the support group was the sharing amongst group members.

The general style of the New Haven ECaP groups was different from that of the Charlie Brown support group described in the next section. Fees were charged on a sliding scale (no one was ever turned away for financial reasons) since the group leaders were paid professionals. There was an intake interview, and the groups were generally limited to 12 people (guests were welcome) and a fixed number of meetings. There was a significant psychotherapy orientation to the sessions, music was often used, and drawings were encouraged. There were separate groups for people with a life-challenging disease, HIV/AIDS, and caregivers. Hugging was always important. People were focused on changing their lives, since these were not 'victim' groups. The overall atmosphere was of a warm and caring place.

3.4 The Charlie Brown Exceptional Patient Support Group (Dayton)

The group was started by Charlie Flynn after he 'graduated' from hospice. After he read Bernie Siegel's first book while a patient in hospice with a short life expectancy, he decided he liked Bernie's philosophy, and that he wasn't going to die of cancer. His cancer went into remission and Charlie walked out. With the help of his surgeon, Dr. George Brown, and several professionals, the Charlie Brown group was launched in October of 1990. Charlie died three years later on Christmas Eve of a heart attack, but his group continues.

Since the people who attend this group find it particularly helpful, the important features will be described in some detail to help you establish a similar group. The group is open to anyone who has a life-challenging disease and supporters. Sometimes, it is just the support person who attends. There are no fees. The group meets twice monthly year-round for one and one-half hours. There is a free lending library. Refreshments are always available.

There are a few rules—perhaps the most important one is confidentiality. The expectation is that anything said in the room stays there. Each person gets a chance to talk, and he can talk for as long as he wishes. Interruptions or comments are not permitted—each person talks until he is done. The expectation is that everyone else gives the speaker their undivided, respectful, and caring attention. Even if there is time after everyone has spoken, commenting (asking questions or offering advice, for example) is not permitted during this time. After the meeting is over, people do talk to each other and share in a private manner. The leaders do not comment, interrupt, or offer suggestions. We start and end the meeting, do the healing meditation at the end, and chair the non-sharing portions of the meeting. The healing power of the group lies in the unconditional respectful attention everyone gets. This is often the only place where you can really speak from your heart, and share whatever is within you.

The order of a typical meeting starts with hugs on entering—there is even an official 'chief hugger.' Everyone wears a name tag with

Figure 3.1: A support group meeting.

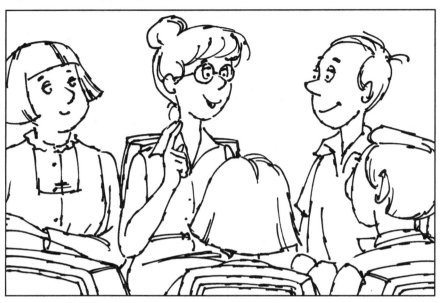

their first name in large letters. We always sit in a circle so everyone can see all of the people at the meeting. One of the leaders of the group calls the meeting to order and, if there is a new member present, relates the history and purpose of group. The operating rules are also repeated. New members get a list of our operating rules, a flyer, a hug card, and an address list. If there are any business or announcements, they are handled rapidly. Next, we ask for updates on members who are not present. At that time we decide who gets a hope/healing/we're-thinking-of-you card. These are circulated along with an attendance sheet. Everyone is expected to write a few encouraging words or greetings, whether or not they know the addressee. We are then ready for sharing time. One of the leaders decides the direction of the order of speaking so that new members get to speak later in the meeting. If there is time after all have spoken, then anyone can enlarge or add to their own *personal* statement.

The meeting ends with dimming the lights and moving the chairs so everyone can hold hands in a large circle. One of the leaders then does a healing meditation that lasts for five to 10 minutes. This healing meditation usually weaves into its content some theme or themes of the day or of the meeting itself. The meditation always ends with the *Serenity Prayer*:

> (God) grant me the serenity to accept the things I cannot change, the courage to change the things I can, and the wisdom to know the difference. (Amen)

The lights are raised, hugs are available for those who want them, and people chat with each other for a few minutes. This kind of group can be an instrument of healing, and members become quite loyal.

3.5 Residential and other Support Groups

There are a number of residential support groups for people who have life-challenging diseases that admit patients for typically one week. Fink's book (1997) *Third Opinion* is, as its subtitle states, "An international directory to alternative therapy centers for the treatment and prevention of cancer and other degenerative diseases." In addition to these residential centers, Fink also gives information about alternative treatment programs worldwide. A brief description is given for each entry, along with contact information and estimated costs. Lerner (1996) has an extensive appendix with names and contact information for alternative therapy programs.

Perhaps the two best-known residential programs are Commonweal (Lerner is its director and Rachel Naomi Remen, M.D., is its medical director. Their address is: P.O. Box 316, Bolinas, CA 94924; (415) 868-0970) and the Simonton Cancer Center (O. Carl Simonton, M.D., is the director. Simonton Cancer Center, P.O. Box 890, Pacific Palisades, CA 90272; (800) 459-3424). There are other centers and programs, but they all need to be checked or visited to find out if that is the right program for you.

The Wellness Community (2716 Ocean Park Blvd., Suite 1040, Santa Monica, CA 90405; (310) 314-2555) is a national, free support group with chapters in many locations. The American Cancer Society sponsors support groups in many cities and is a good source of information (1599 Clifton Road, N.E., Atlanta, GA 30329; (800) 227–2345). The National Cancer Institute of NIH has an informational hotline (800-4-CANCER) and a website (www.nci.nih.gov). Also see Appendix B for some relevant websites and phone numbers.

Chapter Four
Journaling, Structured Writing, Videotaping, Art Therapy, and Ceremonies

4.1 Introduction

Guided imagery and psychotherapy-based approaches are just two of many and varied procedures that are helpful to people who have life-challenging diseases. There are a number of adjunctive activities that people can do to help them during the particularly stressful times of diagnosis, treatments, hospitalizations, and in-between periods. Bernie Siegel's third book (1993) is entitled *How To Live Between Office Visits.* (Also see his other three books: Siegel, 1986, 1989, 1998.) What do you do with all that in-between time? Are there things that ease the day or add meaning to your life? In this chapter, a number of useful activities are discussed.

4.2 Journaling

Many people have kept a daily diary at some point in their lives. This practice was more prevalent years ago than at the present time. Sometimes journals are kept for specific purposes like: (1) recording details of a vacation trip; (2) listing amounts and types of all food ingested; (3) listing all physical activity; (4) noting the time, intensity, location, and quality of pain; and (5) noting all medications. But mostly, journals are kept as a personal log of feelings, ideas, observations, and activities.

A diagnosis of cancer, or some other life-challenging disease, immediately raises thoughts of mortality and the meaning of one's life. What is it all about? Why me? Why now? Why this particular disease? Lots and lots of questions bedevil you. It almost seems like an unfair double tragedy to be forced prematurely into considering these questions at a time of great emotional and physical distress. The big 'Why' questions need time and undistracted thinking to work through.

The practice of regularly writing in a journal can be helpful. A person with a life-challenging disease is considered by many to be 'abnormal' in the sense of not being in a normal healthy state. Many friends and relatives find it awkward to communicate with them. Some people just won't or can't listen. There are others who do— you can usually rely on some professionals such as social workers and psychotherapists. But, *you* can write anything as often as you wish in your private journal. No one judges what is written—the deepest innermost thoughts are safe. Most people find journaling to be cathartic. Many people include drawings in their journals. If it is difficult to write, an alternative is to audiotape a journal. Journaling helps in a variety of ways. Just the act of recording, writing from your heart, has beneficial effects. It is a chance to let out your feelings, your fears, your hopes, your dreams. It is a way to bring some order and meaning into your life. It provides connections with your past, as well as your hopes for the future. The very act of writing is frequently a release, and can bring a sense of being in charge. Please consider journaling.

Figure 4.1: Writing in your journal.

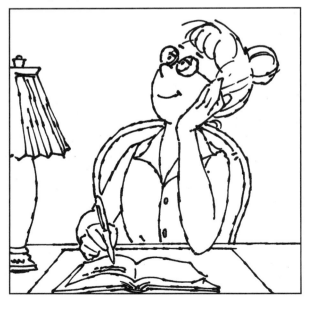

4.3 Structured Writing—A Workbook for People who have Cancer or other Life-Challenging Disease

Structured writing is different from keeping a journal or a diary. The writer answers specific questions designed to help solve a particular problem or deal with a specific condition. There is much evidence that writing about traumatic events can help you minimize their impact on your life. To give you some sense about how this may work for a life-challenging disease, this section presents a 'workbook' for anyone who has been diagnosed with cancer or other life-challenging disease. No systematic evaluation has yet been done of this workbook, but it has been developed with feedback and commentary from a number of people who have different kinds of cancer. Although the following workbook was initially developed with people who have cancer, it can be used without change for other serious diseases like AIDS, diabetes, and many of the chronic neurological diseases. (The workbook may be freely copied and used. I would appreciate receiving feedback on its utility and how to improve it.)

Workbook for People who have Cancer or other Life-Challenging Disease

The questions in this workbook have been designed to help you cope with a diagnosis of cancer or other life-challenging disease, and with its treatment. Please find a quiet time and place to do this writing over a period of successive days (or whenever you are up to doing this kind of writing). What you write is personal and should be kept private. It is your decision about sharing any part of this, or all of it, with someone you trust. If you need more than the allotted space, please continue your responses on the back of the paper or on separate sheets. There are no 'correct' responses— whatever you write is the right thing for you. Take whatever time you need to respond. Many people find that the very act of writing responses to the kinds of questions in this workbook has been helpful in resolving painful concerns. (Within the framework of this book, there is really no room on the pages to respond to these questions—write your answers in a notebook or on a note pad. You can reproduce the table in Question Five for ease of answering.)

1. Use the following space to respond to these three related questions. You may not be able to answer them with any certainty— in that case, you may have a guess or a theory about how to answer the questions.
   a. Why is this happening to me (versus someone else)?
   b. Why is this happening to me at this particular time of my life?
   c. Why do I have this particular kind of cancer or disease?
2. Do you know, or do you have a theory, or can you guess as to why at this particular time you are doing better, or worse, or staying the same?
3. What ways of taking care of yourself are you waiting to explore? (These can be things like: second or third opinions, more research on available medical treatments, alternative or complementary treatments, support groups, support networks, or personal things like counseling/psychotherapy.)
4. What is stopping you from exploring the options in (3) now? What resources do you need to be able to do whatever is necessary to help yourself in (3)?
5. This question has to do with being able to communicate openly about your condition, and your feelings about this condition, with the people in your life. Think carefully about whom you can talk to about the following items, listing *specific* people in each row (for example, you may write in the name of a particular cousin in the row for relatives). For your guidance, there are a number of general categories of people listed in the first column. In each box, put a '+' if you would feel comfortable talking with them about that item, a '-' if this would be a mistake and they would be unresponsive, and a '?' if you are unsure of their responsiveness. Feel free to write additional comments in each box. Where there is more than one person in a category (like friends), please list them separately.

I can talk to this person about …

People	Physical feelings	Emotional feelings	Fears	Spiritual matters	Treatments	Information	Financial matters	Fun and relaxation
Spouse								
Children								
Parents								
Relatives								
Friends								
Doctors								
Counselor								
God								
Minister								
People at work								
Support group								

6. Take some time to write about your fears—your fears for yourself, your family, and your future.

7. Take some time to write about your hopes and dreams, and what it is you would like to do with the remainder of your life. What are the things that you always wanted to do? Which of them can you do now? If and when your health improves, what are the things that you would be sure to do?

8. Write about your feelings about surgery, radiation, chemotherapy, and any other medical treatments.

9. Some surgeries (like mastectomies and prostatectomies) involve the loss of body parts, particularly those that are related to body- and self-image. Please use this space to write about your feelings concerning such surgery (if you have undergone one).

10. Write about your feelings about being in a hospital.

11. Write about your feelings about dealing with medical personnel. Was anyone particularly helpful or difficult?

12. Write about what frustrates you about your particular disease.

13. It is not unusual for people who have been diagnosed with cancer or some other serious ailment to have the seemingly paradoxical reaction of considering it to be a 'blessing' in some way. What things have you learned about yourself and about the people around you that are beneficial to you?

14. How has having this serious disease changed your spiritual life?

15. Knowing what you know now about your life, if you could, how would you have lived differently? That is, what would you change about your past life?

16. Knowing what you know now about your life, what things will you do differently starting right now?

17. Sometimes opportunities for saying things to people just bypass us. Are there significant people in your past whom you never had a chance to tell what was really on your mind or in your heart? Write what you would have told them if you had the chance. (These people may be living or dead.)

18. This is related to 17. Write out what things for your spouse and children (or specific others) you want to: (a) have them know; (b) leave them (personal items or thoughts); and (c) say to them. You may wish to share these writings with them now, later, leave the writings for them, or continue to keep them private.

19. Although this is a trying time, it is always wise to take care of certain 'mechanical' things like wills, living wills, durable power of attorney for health, financial matters, and funeral

arrangements as soon as possible. Most people make these arrangements when they are well and not faced with difficult times. Once taken care of, you no longer need to be concerned about them. If you have not already done so, make appointments to take care of these items. This space would also be a good place to write about your feelings about these items. (*Note*: This item may be difficult to handle at this time, and you may wish to put it off for a while and/or discuss it with someone you trust. Many people in good health attend to these items in healthy times just so there would be no surprises or difficulties for their children or other family members. They also regularly review these items. But please respond to this item only when you feel comfortable about doing so.)

20. Write about anything else that concerns you at this time. This is *your private* journal and you can write whatever you wish.

4.4 Structured Writing—A Workbook for Grieving

One of life's major traumas is the death of a spouse, a family member, or someone you are very close to. Writing and talking about the death (see Pennebaker, 1987, pp. 20–25, 73–88) really helps. In fact, the more you do this, the fewer health problems you will have. Prayer is actually one way of 'talking.' It turns out that the ways you write or talk about upsetting experiences are important. It helps to explore your deepest thoughts and feelings in a reflective way. Some people feel a bit sad or depressed immediately after writing, but these feelings quickly go away and give way to a sense of lasting relief.

Writing for grieving is in two parts. The *first* involves just setting aside time to write continuously about your deepest thoughts and feelings for 20 to 30 minutes for several days. Then, return to this style of writing periodically, perhaps once a month, as you feel the need to put your thoughts down. The *second* part involves the structured writing in the following workbook. If you write for yourself, that is, you do not intend to show what you have written to anyone else, then the writing is more effective since you can be more honest and open. It may be weeks or months before you feel comfortable in doing personal writing or answering the questions in the workbook. Write in your own way and at your own pace and in your own time.

Workbook for Grievers

The questions in this workbook have been designed to help you cope with a traumatic loss. Please find a quiet time and place to do this writing over a period of successive days or whenever you feel comfortable responding to the questions. What you write is personal and should be kept private. It is your decision about sharing any part of this, or all of it, with someone you trust. If you need more than the allotted space, please continue your responses on the back of the paper or on separate sheets. There are no 'correct' responses—whatever you write is the right thing for you. Take whatever time you need to respond. You should know that a number of research studies have shown that the very act of writing responses to the kinds of questions in this workbook has been beneficial for both physical and mental health. (There is obviously not room to write answers in this book. Please write responses in a notebook or notepad. You can reproduce the table in Question Seven.)

1. Write in detail about the good times you had with the person whose loss you are grieving.
2. Write about losses that you shared and experienced together.
3. What special personal characteristics will see you through this time?
4. What are your special strengths?
5. What ways of taking care of yourself are you willing to explore at this time? How will you overcome things that are in the way of you taking care of yourself?
6. What is different about the times when you are able to function normally? How can you extend those times?
7. Whom can you communicate with openly about your loss and your feelings? Think carefully about whom you can talk to about the items in the table, listing *specific* people in each row (for example, in the row marked relatives you might list a particular cousin). (You can add more rows if needed.) Mark boxes with a '+' if you feel comfortable talking with them about that item, a '-' if this is a mistake and they would be unresponsive or unhelpful, and a '?' if you are unsure about their responsiveness. You may write additional comments in each box.

People	Physical feelings	Emotional feelings	Fears	Spiritual matters	Memories	Loneliness	Hopes and dreams
Spouse							
Children							
Parents							
Relatives							
Friends							
Doctors							
Counselor							
God							
Minister							
People at work							
Support group							

I can talk to this person about …

8.   Write about fears—and your fears for yourself, for your family, and for your future.

9.   Write about your hopes and dreams, and what it is you would like to do with the rest of your life. What are the things that you always wanted to do? When will you do them?

10.   Write about how this loss has changed your life. How do you plan to adapt to or overcome these changes and go on with your life?

11.   How has this loss affected your spiritual life?

12.   How has this loss affected your social life? Relationships with your family? Friends? Acquaintances? Fellow workers?

13.   Sometimes opportunities to say things to people bypass us. Are there significant people in your past that you never had a chance to tell what was really on your mind or in your heart? Write what you would have told them if you had the chance. The people you write to in this workbook may be gone or still alive—in particular, it may be the person you've just lost.

14.   Use the following space to write about anything else that concerns you at this time. This is *your private* journal and you can write whatever you wish.

4.5 Structured Writing—A Workbook for Caregivers

Caregivers are the unsung heroes and heroines taking care of loved ones who have life-challenging diseases. Bernie Siegel has commented about families visiting his office: he observed that the person who appeared to be under the least stress was the person with the active ailment. She knew what was wrong within her body and had already come to terms with it in some way. It was her family who were worried and tense and anxious, not knowing what to expect or how to cope.

Who cares for the caregivers; who helps the helpers? Taking care of someone you love through the months and years of cancer, or the years of Alzheimer's disease, or other serious diseases is exceedingly stressful. Yet, somehow, people call on hidden reserves of energy and strength and compassion to survive these ordeals. There are many support groups for people with named diseases, but many fewer for caregivers.

This workbook has been designed specifically for caregivers, to lead them through a series of writings that provide an outlet for all of those unexpressed inner feelings and questions and tensions. Again, keeping the writing private makes it easier to 'write from the heart.' Caregivers, like survivors, need to let go of the regrets of the past and the fear of the future and learn to live in the present— one day at a time. Some themes that arise may become the basis for discussions with a trusted person.

Workbook for Caregivers

The questions in this workbook have been designed to help you as a caregiver cope with the stress of being a caregiver. Please find a quiet time and place to do this writing over a period of successive days. What you write is personal and should be kept private. It is your decision about sharing any part of this, or all of it, with some- one you trust. If you need more than the allotted space, please con- tinue your responses on the back of the paper or on separate sheets. There are no 'correct' responses—whatever you write is the right thing for you. Take whatever time you need to respond. The very act of writing responses to the kinds of questions in this workbook has been beneficial for both physical and mental health. This process is most helpful when you 'write from the heart.'

1. The following three questions are related. You may not be able to answer them with certainty—in that case, you may have a guess or a theory about how to answer these questions
   a. Why is this happening to the person I love (versus someone else)?
   b. Why is this happening to him/her at this particular time?
   c. Why does he/she have this particular disease (versus a different one)?
2. Do you know, or do you have a theory, or can you guess why he/she is doing better, or worse, or staying the same at this time?
3. Write in detail about the good times you have had with the per- son for whom you are caring.
4. Write about special memories or experiences the two of you have shared.

5. Write about losses that you have shared and experienced together.
6. What special personal characteristics will see you through this time?
7. What are your special strengths?
8. What additional ways of taking care of yourself are you willing to explore at this time? How will you overcome things that are in the way of you taking care of yourself?
9. What ways can you share the work of caring? Who can help? Can you set up a network of helpers or have someone do this for you?
10. It is not unusual to feel anger and frustration, sometimes about the person for whom you are caring. There can even be occasional thoughts about wishing it were all over already. If you are experiencing any of these emotions, here is a private place to write.
11. Write about your fears—your fears for yourself, for your family, for your future.
12. Write about how these circumstances have changed your life. How do you plan to adapt to or overcome these changes and go on with your life?
13. How have these circumstances affected your spiritual life?
14. How has your involvement with caregiving affected your relationship with the person you are caring for? Relationships with your family? Friends? Acquaintances? Social life? Work life?
15. Are there things you would like to tell the person you are caring for at this time? When will you make an opportunity to do that? On the other hand, there may be things that you would prefer to write rather than speak—do that here.
16. Sometimes, opportunities to say things to people bypass us. Are there other significant people in your past that you never had a chance to tell what was really on your mind or in your heart? Write what you would have told them if you had the chance. The people you write to in this section may be gone or still alive.
17. Whom can you communicate with openly about being a caregiver, about your feelings? Think carefully about whom you can talk to about the items in the following table, listing *specific* people in each row (for example, in the row marked relatives you might list a particular cousin). (You can add more rows if needed.) Mark boxes with a '+' if you feel comfortable talking with them about that item, a '-' if this is a mistake and they would be unresponsive

I can talk to this person about …

People	Physical feelings	Emotional feelings	Fears	Spiritual matters	Memories	Loneliness	Hopes and dreams
Spouse							
Children							
Parents							
Relatives							
Friends							
Doctors							
Counselor							
God							
Minister							
People at work							
Support group							

or unhelpful, and a '?' if you are unsure about their responsiveness. You may write additional comments in each box.

18. Although this is a trying time, it is always wise to take care of certain 'mechanical' things like wills, living wills, durable power of attorney for health care, financial matters, and funeral arrangements as soon as possible. Most people make these arrangements when they are well and not faced with difficult times. Once taken care of, you no longer need to be concerned about them. If you have not already done so, make appointments to take care of these items. This space would also be a good place to write about your feelings about these items. (*Note*: This item may be difficult to handle at this time, and you may wish to put it off for a while and/or discuss it with someone you trust. Many people in good health attend to these items in advance, just so there will be no surprises or difficulties for their children or others. They also regularly review these items. Please respond to this item only when you feel comfortable doing so.)

19. You may think that it is premature to write about your hopes and dreams, and what it is you would like to do with the rest of *your* life. Yet, this may be an appropriate time. If it is, what are the things that you always wanted to do? When will you do them?

20. Use the following space to write about anything else that concerns you at this time. This is *your private* journal and you can write whatever you wish.

4.6 Videotaping and Autobiographies

Rainwater (1979) has written of her experience with geriatric clients with respect to the importance of telling their life stories. In the telling (and retelling) of the stories of one's life, there is a self-validation that appears to be most comforting and reassuring for older people. This is particularly true for people of any age who face foreshortened lives due to disease or accident. The very act of telling or writing about one's life, history, activities, achievements (and even failures) brings that life into perspective, roots it in history, and gives it value and meaning. It is almost a discovering of "Oh, I didn't realize how much I had done, all the places I've been, all the lives I've touched and whose lives have touched mine, the significance of some of these little things, those magic moments I had forgotten, the specialness of ordinary living." You might recall that most poignant cemetery scene in Thornton Wilder's *Our Town,* in which Emily discovers the importance, the magic, of everyday life growing up in Grover's Corners. We all need this appreciation of the mundane, if you will, to find out what is really important in life, what has been really important in our past, and what can be important in our current day-to-day lives if we only look.

Recording your life by writing an autobiography is one way to attain this perspective and validation. Two of my friends have done this: one had colorectal cancer (he died in 1997), and the other has many life problems associated with adult onset diabetes and renal failure which requires thrice weekly dialysis. For my former friend, the autobiography was for family and friends. The surviving friend's biography is for friends, professional colleagues, and other interested people. It was the *act* of writing that was important for them— polishing the words was unimportant. If you write an autobiography, be sure to raise the question of who will be your intended audience. It is certainly okay if there is no intended audience, and directions are left to destroy the manuscript upon your death.

If writing is not your thing, or is difficult for you for any reason, then you can explore having a family member or friend make an audiotape or videotape interview of you telling your life story. These tapes will be a heritage for your family and friends. You can make these tapes at any time. The following paragraphs are instructions meant for the person doing the videotaping.

A two-hour videotape is about the right length of time. The person being taped should set the pace and length of sessions. Sometimes, the tape is done in one session, and sometimes two. Typically, the interviewee says she can think of only a few things to say, maybe for ten or fifteen minutes. Yet, once she gets started, she will forget the camera and the time. If she does not wish to be seen on camera, suggest that you will not focus on her face, but just focus on hands or objects in the room. She may want to include furniture or knick-knacks or photographs or mementoes of special interest.

It is helpful to have someone lead the person through their life, starting with when and where they were born, information about

Figure 4.2: Videotaping a life history.

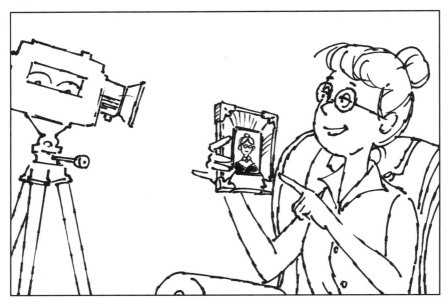

their parents, where they grew up, how and when they met, where they lived, and their occupations. What are some of their earliest memories? Any siblings? What was it like as a child, pre-teen, teen, young adult? What was their social life? How did they meet and fall in love with their spouse? (When interviewing a husband and wife, elicit this information separately to the point of their marriage.) What was their early married life like? Bringing up children? Occupations and avocations? Travels? Grown children and grand-parenting? Any special advice for children and grandchildren? The ending is "Anything else you'd like to say?" Then, thank them for the privilege of hearing about their life.

Mechanical aspects need attention. If at all possible, everyone should be 'miked.' Lighting is not too important because modern videocameras have extraordinary light sensitivity. They all have zoom and autofocus features. To make the tape less static, vary the frame from long shots to close-ups. If it is appropriate, use the fade-in and fade-out feature. When using the zoom feature, be sure to change the frame *slowly*. Also, any panning should be done slowly. Record the data and time vocally as well as with those built-in features in the camera. The camera should be mounted on a sturdy tripod. As the interviewer, do not stay glued behind the camera, but change the zoom, move to the side, and move behind the camera only to make adjustments at intervals. If you have a second person run the camera, that makes the interviewing easier. Editing of the tapes is generally not done. Keep the original and make as many copies for family and friends as the interviewee requests. There are many hospice units that provide a loaner videocamera for the use of family members. If you do not own a videocamera, borrow one from a friend or rent one.

4.7 Art Therapy

Drawing can sometimes be quite helpful. You do not need to be an artist to do this. Just draw what comes to your mind in whatever way(s) you can. A set of colored felt-tipped pens are useful for this purpose. Drawings can be just relaxing, or a way to get your innermost feelings on paper. Sometimes a professional therapist can help you with the drawings. They are for you.

Figure 4.3: Drawing for yourself.

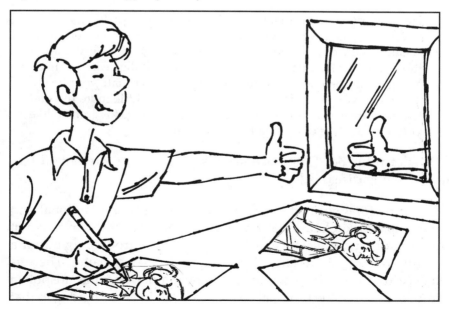

If you are willing, it is helpful to do four drawings. They are: (1) a picture of you as you are now, in your present state or condition;

(2) a drawing of your treatment(s) and/or what you are doing for yourself; (3) a drawing of you after this is over and you are in good health; and (4) how you got from the (1)-present condition to the (3)-full health state. Please note that drawing (4) may be very different from the treatments in (2). You may wish to title and date the drawings. You may also add narratives to the back of the drawings, and give voice to elements of the drawings by adding balloons (as in comic strips). Drawings may be repeated at regular intervals. You can do these four kinds of drawings for yourself or share them with someone.

4.8 *Cancer or other Serious Disease as a Gift*

Cancer as a gift—what a strange, seemingly paradoxical idea! Yet it is not uncommon for people who have a life-challenging disease to make this statement, or something similar. One person said, "You know, before I was diagnosed with prostate cancer I did not know what love was." Scott Hamilton, the ice skating champion who had testicular cancer, has said (Hamilton, 1999):

> I feel almost fortunate that I had that experience in my life, as clearly devastating as it was. I feel like I'm a richer, deeper person for it. Dealing with cancer and the treatment and the recovery and all those things can adjust your outlook on life and the beauty of it all. You get kind of a new lease on life, and you appreciate your health more than you ever did before. Birthdays are a little more fun and holidays are really special and you don't take things for granted like you once did. It's a blessing that I had cancer.

How can this be? [This section uses 'cancer' to represent *all* life-challenging diseases.]

The initial diagnosis of cancer is almost always an emotional and physical shock. Occasionally, it is a relief to have the symptoms of discomfort and malaise, which may have been troubling you for a considerable time, finally diagnosed and given a name. There is relief due to the disappearance of uncertainty and the unspoken implication that the physical condition is 'all in your mind.' Yet that initial shock for most people leads to profound soul-searching. Why me? Why now? Why this? What do I do with the remainder of my life? How much longer do I have to live? Will I suffer? If there is suffering, am I capable of bearing it? Who am I? What am I? Was this predestined? What can I do now?

All of a sudden, life becomes predictably finite. Cancer kills. Can you really believe that cancer is just a word and not a sentence? Invariably, the diagnosis leads to changes in lifestyle. The treatments necessitate much of this. The questionings and re-evaluations lead to more profound changes. With a finite life expectancy, what is really important? Is it that promotion? A new car or house or...? A trip? A raise in pay? That status your ambition drove you towards? What you were going to do after retirement?

The gift of cancer seems to be the recognition of the preciousness of this moment, this breath, this touch or smile or hug, this bite of food, being able to swallow or go to the toilet by yourself, a blade of grass, a cumulus cloud, a raindrop, a glass of cold water on a hot day, a mug of hot cocoa on a cold day, some special music, quiet, serious talking, loving and being loved, a minute of no pain and of no nausea—each moment becomes precious. Suddenly, you recognize how much of your life was hum-drum, routine, automatic, habitual, controlled. Now, you have permission by virtue of your disease to break out of that mold, that prison of musts and shoulds and can'ts. Suddenly, somehow, you become more alive, really live in the moment, tasting and touching and smelling and hearing and looking and being. It is almost like waking up from the dream of unknowingly passing through life, to being aware of each and every thing inside and outside of yourself. You are finally alive, being born to heightened awareness. That is the gift, and people respond to this new awareness with a certain kind of awe. They know that they are different from other people because of the cancer; they also perceive all of those other cancer-free people as somehow flawed, as living inside an insensate shell. Paradoxical? Perhaps. Are they denying the disease? No. They are instead becoming truly realistic in valuing and recognizing reality moment by moment. People who have had 'near-death' experiences react the same way.

You do not need a serious disease to have 'permission' to do the things you've always wanted to do. Just think about the gift of this moment, this breath. Someone has said that the *present* is called that because it really is a present, a gift. And it is a gift that is so obvious that most of us never notice it. The stars at night. Lightning. A sunflower. A hug ...

Figure 4.4a&b: Cancer as a gift.

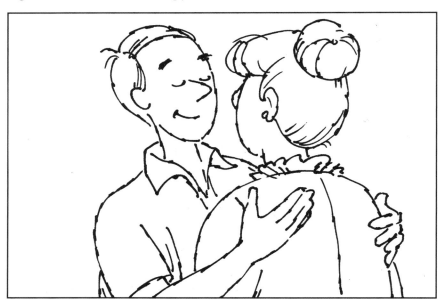

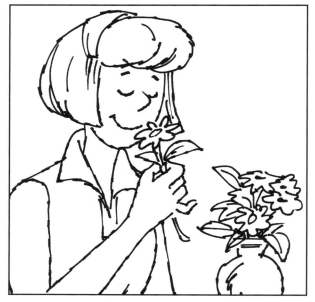

Sharp and Terbay, who both work at Hospice of Dayton, have compiled a book (1997) entitled *Gifts* which is full of stories about people and their gifts. Rachel Naomi Remen's compilation of poetry

(1994) is about gifts. Her book *Kitchen Table Wisdom* (1996) is about the gift of her life. Her latest book, *My Grandfather's Blessings* (2000), is itself a blessing.

What does a person who has been admitted to a hospice program, with a best-guess life expectancy of less than six months, do when her cancer disappears and she 'graduates' from hospice? (This is a rare occurrence, but it does happen.) My friend Claudia graduated from hospice over three years ago. She and her family were realistic—they had even together planned her funeral service. Coming back to life had its difficulties for Claudia and her husband and family and friends. She and her husband continue to live one day at a time. Claudia does volunteer work at hospice and local hospitals. She is sharing her gift. *You* don't need to be a hospice graduate to share your gift of life.

4.9 *Rituals and Ceremonies*

With people who have life-challenging diseases, ceremonies can be constructed for completing unfinished business, ending old and unneeded feelings, or for marking the end of chemotherapy or radiation treatments. Generally, ceremonies are developed in conjunction with family members, and carried out by the family. The power of ceremonies is related to the specificity of the symbols and symbolic actions. Ceremonies are invariably realistic. Some traditions invoke angels, spirit guides and helpers, and power animals. The astute therapist always serves as a guide and resource, working within the client's belief systems and doing things respectfully within those belief systems. There are many different kinds of ceremonies.

Carl Hammerschlag, M.D., tells a remarkable story about his journey from his medical training as a know-it-all New Yorker to working in the Indian (Native American) Service in Arizona to becoming a healer. His story is recounted in two books (1988, 1993) and inspiring audiotapes available through Hammerschlag Ltd. (3104 East Camelback Road, Suite 614, Phoenix, AZ 85016). His personal story goes from traditional Western medicine to healing, from doctor to healer. The subject of this section, however, is based on his book with Silverman (1997) on the use of rituals and ceremonies for healing.

First, Silverman and Hammerschlag make a distinction between rituals and ceremonies. *Rituals* are more like habits in the sense that they are repetitive and become incorporated into daily living. Morning rituals may be the order in which you toilet, shower, dress, shave or put on makeup, have coffee, fold towels, and put on underwear left-foot or right-foot first. These are routine actions that may or may not have had their origins as part of special religious, cultural, or spiritual practices.

Ceremonies, on the other hand, have a connection to the spiritual or sacred or religious, and are special events. Brushing your teeth in a particular way is a ritual, getting married is a ceremony. Succinctly, rituals are routine and ceremonies are special. Ceremonies typically incorporate the following elements:

(1) leader to facilitate
(2) specific goal
(3) significant or sacred object
(4) group of selected people
(5) particular site
(6) mutual respect/reverence
(7) special timing
(8) specific order of service or components

For example, a Western-culture wedding ceremony includes a minister or rabbi, the wedding contract, wedding rings, relatives and friends of the bride and bridegroom, a church or synagogue or hall, an awe and respect of the event itself, a specific date and times for the ceremony and celebration, and an order of service prescribed by the religion, or by the bride and bridegroom.

In the rest of this section, we will give details about: (1) Hammerschlag and Silverman's healing circle; (2) Rachel Naomi Remen's preparation for a medical intervention circle; and (3) ceremonies designed for a specific purpose. Before doing this, however, the elements of the *Navajo Talking Circle*, which are common to many ceremonies, will be described.

Native American Talking Circle. The *Native American Talking Circle* incorporates the eight elements described above. There is a person who is the focus of the circle and her healing may be the

Figure 4.5: A healing circle.

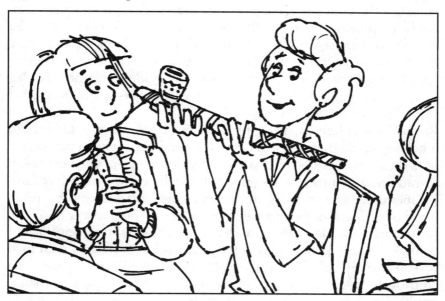

objective of the meeting. She supplies a sacred object, which is passed around the circle. You may talk only when you are holding the object. When you finish, you pass the object on. The rules are: (1) whatever is said and shared in the circle is confidential and not repeated outside; (2) each person talks about her own *personal* experience, from her own heart, for as long as she wishes; (3) when she finishes, the next person has the attention of the group; (4) there is *no* cross-chatter, interruption, or commenting on what others have said; and (5) everyone listens attentively and respectfully to whoever is speaking. For non-Native American groups, a sacred object that is passed around is optional. In the *Native American Talking Circle*, each person speaks only once. In other groups, time permitting, a person may speak again, but only from her own personal perspective—no comments on others or by others—but, perhaps adding something she forgot to say the first time.

Hammerschlag and Silverman have facilitated many healing circles. Their book (1997) gives examples. They traditionally use a sacred object that is passed around, and incorporate the elements mentioned above, as well as the rules for speaking in a *Native American Talking Circle*. The leader acts as organizer and facilitator. At the beginning, the leader explains the purpose of the meeting and the rules. At the end, she closes the meeting, perhaps with some summary comments. The significance of the sacred object may be explained. Participants are specifically invited. They sit in a circle on chairs or on the floor. Lighting is controlled and may include candles or a fire. A sense of the sacred is evident. Hammerschlag says, "When you speak from the heart, you always speak the truth."

Rachel Naomi Remen, M.D. (pp. 151–153, 1996), gives details about a healing circle that is specifically designed to prepare a person for a medical intervention such as surgery or a series of chemotherapy or radiation treatments. The group typically comprises a few family members and friends, and is convened for this sole purpose. They meet a few days or a week or so before the intervention. The central person brings along a small stone that is important to her symbolically. The stone is generally flat and no larger than an inch or so. The central person does not speak, but silently hands the stone to a person seated adjacent to them. *Navajo Talking Circle* rules apply. The person holding the stone tells about some traumatic or difficult event in her life. She then describes what personal characteristic(s) or action(s) helped her through that time. These characteristics are things like: courage, prayer, belief in a Divine Being, persistence, faith, determination, and love. This speech is concluded with "I put *strength* into this stone so you may have it with you" and pass the stone on. Each person ends her tale with a similar statement, endowing the stone with her way or coping and surviving. At the end, the stone, which is imbued with all of these personal gifts, is given to the central person. She tapes the stone to her wrist or palm or foot, and informs the medical staff about its sacred significance. This special healing/preparation ceremony has been used by Remen for over 20 years. In her experience it is quite helpful—she has also received positive feedback from surgeons in her area.

Chapter Five
Varieties of Coping

5.1 *Introduction*

When a person is diagnosed with a life-challenging disease, he enters a whole new world from his normal everyday existence. There are new priorities and demands, which seemingly cannot be postponed or scheduled for his convenience. Appointments for visiting doctors and getting treatments and being tested have to be made and kept. All other day-to-day tasks must be re-scheduled around the appointments. If a surgery or surgeries are involved, then there are hospital stays and recuperation periods. There are changed and changing relationships with family and friends. There are the hard realities of finance and insurance and employment. There may be things like a changing body identity to adjust to in the case of mastectomies or colostomies or amputations, or just a decreased capacity to do everyday things like walking, going up and down stairs, playing sports, taking a shower, or going to the toilet. And most important are the emotional ups and downs, the fears, the anxieties, the hopelessness and helplessness, the depression, the threat of death, the endless 'why' questions, and the sense of unreality that seems to preclude everything else. You have just been forced to step through the looking glass into a dream world that operates with its own strange rules. How do you cope? How do your family and friends cope?

This chapter is a collection of many things about coping. It is written both for patients and caregivers. Patients and caregivers will find many practical ways to cope.

For your guidance this paragraph lists a number of sources on the subject of coping. LeShan's 1989 book contains an excellent chapter (pp. 80–100) on dealing with hospitals and the medical establishment. This is summarized in the next section. The American Cancer Society and the National Cancer Institute of the NIH have free pamphlets on coping, as do support groups for other diseases.

Appendix B lists a number of websites and contains useful phone numbers. Milstein's book (1994), *Giving Comfort, What You Can Do When Someone You Love Is Ill*, is an excellent compendium of practical coping ideas. In fact, there are over three hundred numbered suggestions in various categories. Unfortunately, this great book is out of print. Some of her suggestions are given in Section 5.3. Doka (1993) has written a comprehensive and resource-full book whose title is descriptive: *Living With Life-Threatening Illness: A Guide for Patients, Their Families & Caregivers*. At the end of this chapter (Section 5.28) is Doka's list of the phases of a life-challenging disease— you may find this to be a useful guide. Doka has written (1993, p. 11), "Life-threatening illness is inevitably family illness, for the life of everyone within the family is changed when one member of a family experiences disease."

5.2 LeShan on How to Survive in a Hospital

Based on his many years of working as a psychologist with the terminally ill in hospital settings, LeShan (1989, pp. 80–100) has much helpful advice to give on how to survive in a hospital. This is summarized in what follows as a series of bulleted items.

- [with respect to hospital philosophy] They define a *good* patient as one who accepts their statements and actions uncritically and unquestioningly. A *bad* patient is one who asks questions to which they do not have the answers, raises problems with which they are uncomfortable, and does not accept hospital procedures as necessarily wise, useful, or intelligent. There is a tremendous pressure on the staff to regard the institution's rules as correct and the individual patient who objects to them as wrong. (p. 81)
- ... if possible have a friend or a relative who can be your advocate. (p. 87)
- Before you enter the hospital, there are certain facts you should have and certain questions you should ask. 1. Who is the physician who has the overall responsibility for your care? 2. What is the diagnosis, and how certain of it is your physician? 3. What is the usual course of the disease, both with and without therapy? 4. What are the side effects of the therapy? 5. What alternatives exist? ... Will the physician's course of action

change depending on the results of the test? *If not, there is no reason to take it....* Remember that the hospital is in the business of selling services, and these include diagnostic tests.... The search for a diagnosis may acquire a life of its own ... The more tests that are performed, the more likely the results of at least one looking unusual. (pp. 88–90)

- When you are speaking to a physician about an illness, keep checking to make sure that you are hearing each other.... Do not let yourself be ignored if there is something that the physician should know or should be paying attention to. The word *no* is powerful.... You must also control the number of people who will give you physical examinations. The resident on service needs to examine you because if anything goes wrong he or she has to make quick decisions and so must know your body from direct examination. Ask your personal physician if there are any other physicians who *must* do this. (pp. 91–92)

- On the pad of paper on your bedside table, have your physician list all of the medications you are supposed to get, at what times you get each, and what each looks like. (p. 92)

- Find out what diet you will be on and whether you can have food brought in from the outside. (p. 92)

Figure 5.1: I'm sorry—you can't examine me.

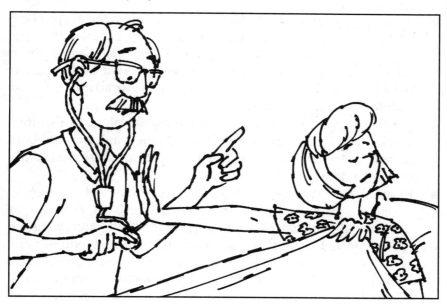

- The charge nurse ... will come in to introduce herself ... if she does not, send her a message that you would like to meet her. (p. 92)
- Feel free to complain. You do not have to be a good child. Complaints will get you better service. (p. 93)
- The Patient's Bill of Rights [also see Appendix C] states in part: *Any competent adult has the absolute right to refuse treatment. Any competent adult has the absolute right to refuse to be examined by any particular individual. Any competent adult has the absolute right to refuse to participate in teaching activities.* (p. 97)
- You also have the right to know the results of all tests made on you ... tell your physician to make a note in your chart and to inform the nursing station that any questions you ask are to be answered.... You also have the right to see your chart any time you wish ... but don't try to read the chart yourself. (pp. 93–94)
- You can leave the hospital at any time.... The hospital may request you to sign an against-medical-advice (AMA) form, but they can only request this and cannot hold you if you refuse. (p. 94)
- Unauthorized medical treatments (except in clear and obvious life-and-death situations) constitute assault and battery.... Consent is the key. (p. 94)
- As far as surgical procedures go, the rule is the less the better. (p. 94)
- Among the things you should carry with you to the hospital are the usual medications you take regularly or occasionally. Ask your regular physician *before you enter the hospital* if any of these are contraindicated by the procedures you will undergo.... If someone tries to take them away, you or your advocate friend should simply forbid it. (p. 96)
- [on your bedside pad] write your personal physician's office and home telephone numbers as well as the name and numbers of any physicians who will have much to do with you while you are a patient ... (p. 96)
- In many hospitals psychiatrists and psychologists are seen as special disciplinary arms of the medical service.... The thing to do when a psychiatrist visits you under these circumstances [not requested by you] is to say politely "I did not request your visit. I will not talk to you. I will refuse any bill you send to me. Please go away." ... If they are too persistent, telephone the hospital administrator and say that there is an unauthorized

person in your room who refuses to leave. That should do the trick. (pp. 96–97)

● By all means take tranquilizers in this situation or others when they are indicated. But you should remain in control of what agents you take to affect your brain. By and large, the more you stay in control of your own destiny, the better you will do. (p. 98)

Wow! What a compendium of useful survival tactics for a hospital stay. Some of the items mentioned above will appear in different contexts throughout the remainder of this chapter.

5.3 Milstein's Coping Suggestions and Comments

Milstein (1994) lists hundreds of practical suggestions for coping. Her book also contains much sound advice for both caregivers and those with an active disease. Since this excellent book is out of print, a number of her suggestions are given in this section. (A number preceding an item corresponds with one of her numbered suggestions.)

1. Show that you care by simply being there.
2. Make short, frequent visits that will not wear you or your loved one out.
3. If she is tired and weak, she may simply like to hear your voice, in person or over the phone, even if she doesn't feel like talking.
4. Help your loved one keep friendships going.
5. Be a friendly listener.
6. Be an honest friend ... there is nothing you can say about your loved one's illness that she hasn't already thought of in private.
17. Listen unreservedly to your loved one's reports of her physical and medical changes and routines.
18. Listen tolerantly to your loved one's anger at old wounds, new hurts, life, the current situation. Listen uncritically to complaints, large and small, real and imagined.
19. Listen bravely to your loved one's fears, worries, and uncertainties.... You cannot truly travel with your loved one on the

road in this illness. But you can accompany this special person in facing her secret concerns.

20. Listen compassionately to your loved one's treatment plans (or plans to refuse treatment).
21. Praise your loved one for all of the good things in her life. Appreciate the positive: her good qualities, friendships, and happy experiences.
22. Forgive your loved one for past grievances.
    - Physical touch is the most important and immediate way to express your feelings for your loved one. (p. 53)
    - It's often easy to lose sight of the person behind the illness. Your loved one may be sick, perhaps quite seriously, but your relationship is with the person, not the illness. (p. 69)
229. ... Ultimately your loved one must die without you. Do not leave him first, emotionally, before he has a chance to leave you in reality.
233. Tolerate. Tolerate your loved one's anger without returning it. Tolerate your loved one's fear without succumbing to it.
    - You cannot stop death, or avoid it, or defeat it, or take your loved one's place in it. You can, however, be alongside your loved one when she dies. Your presence is, and always was, the best comfort you can give. (p. 99)
    - It can be comforting to talk about the hopes and plans that he is not able to fulfill himself, but would want others to continue in his absence. Anticipating the future together can make your loved one feel he has a share in it. (p. 102)
292. Gather strength from your own good health. Take especially good care of your physical condition. Do not ignore little symptoms or neglect routine check-ups and medical and dental care. Do not compare your problems with your loved one's. Your first job is to keep well, so you can do all the other things you want to do.
    - Giving yourself some of the comfort and care you have given your loved one will help restore your capacity to give more in the future. (P. 121)

Milstein emphasizes *listening* and *being there*. Her book is a great collection of useful advice and ideas—the preceding is but a sample.

5.4 Communicating with Medical Personnel

A standard part of the curriculum for medical doctors and nurses is how to communicate with patients. This training includes practice sessions under supervision. It is also fair to say that doctors and nurses enter their professions due to personal ideals about helping people who are physically ill in some way. They typically begin with compassion and concern. Yet, the training of physicians when they are hospital residents involves such incredible physical and mental strains that the system almost forces a mechanical, 'scientific' and 'objective' approach on them. It is not uncommon for a doctor to be on call every other night. Being on call means being on duty, or available for duty, for a continuous thirty-six hour period. The life of a resident involves being tired and sleep-deprived almost all of the time. And this post-M.D. training can go on for up to ten years depending on the specialty. With managed care, the demands on nurses have also multiplied. The system is inadvertently designed to strip away feeling and reduce medical personnel to technicians. The wonder, the real wonder of all of this, is that *most* medical personnel remain compassionate, cheerful, and involved in the welfare of their patients. They are really caring people. The sad part is that a few of these initially idealistic people do get coarsened and remote and mechanical. On the other hand, to be fair, we also have heard doctors and nurses complain about patients who abuse them. This is not physical abuse, but rudeness, disrespect and disregard. Remember that any interaction between you and a doctor or nurse or medical technician is a two-way street. You may not be able to control their behavior, but you should always be able to control your own behavior and reactions. This section is about things *you* can do, that are under your control, in these interactions.

Perhaps the first thing to keep in mind is that, as you are the consumer or purchaser of medical services, *they work for you*. In that sense, you are their boss. One way to think about this is the distinction between the roles of patient and client. Isn't it implied in the word 'patient' that you need to *be patient*, to be passive, to *wait* until you are told what to do or have done to you? Being a patient vis-a-vis a doctor, for example, places you in the 'one-down' position—you are not an equal in any way. Yes, the medical doctor has more knowledge and experience than you do in his field. He should be respected for his knowledge and skill and accomplishment in the same way that a musician, a tailor, a plumber, a chef, a professor, and an experienced hauler of trash (a 'garbologist') need to be respected. Is there an extra aura due to the fact that doctors may be involved in life or death decisions in their work? Yes, this needs to be acknowledged. However, in a similar way, the captain flying a 747 on a transoceanic flight and the driver of a tourist bus in mountainous terrain also have the potential of life and death decisions in their skilled hands.

Think of the relationship this way: a *client* is someone who *hires* the services of a professional. The professional (doctor, lawyer, plumber, electrician, car mechanic) works *for* the client on a fee-for-service basis. **If you can hire a professional, you can also fire him, and you can do this without giving reasons—this is your prerogative as the purchaser, the client.** One of the functions of support groups is to give support to a member who reports unsatisfactory medical services. You are under no obligation to continue with a particular doctor if you are not satisfied with him for whatever reason. Out of politeness, you may tell him that you are considering switching physicians and why. Common reasons are: a doctor who will not answer questions; a doctor who is cold or remote; a doctor whose examination is perfunctory; or a doctor who is inaccessible. Generally, you have choice in your physicians—there are some health plans where this is not the case. If you can't change to another more open plan, then you are stuck and need to work defensively within that system. Appendix C contains a *Patient's Bill of Rights* taken from Siegel (1986, pp. 127–128).

Elaine was in her seventies when she was diagnosed with breast cancer. Her first surgeon/oncologist worked in a nearby hospital. It might have been a plus for Elaine that the hospital was local and that the physician was a woman. Yet, Elaine found her to be cold and unresponsive and overly 'professional.' This physician was 'fired.' Friends then helped Elaine researched physicians within a reasonable area. In the big city, which was 70 minutes away by car, Elaine found her perfect physician. On the initial interview, accompanied by her husband, Elaine said this wonderful doctor spent two and one-half hours doing an examination, answering all of their questions, and describing options. This surgeon did a lumpectomy and nodal dissection and Elaine is still under her care. You have choices.

It is always a good practice to research your disease, and to be prepared with knowledgeable questions at your appointments. Write out the questions and concerns in advance of the appointment. There is nothing wrong with reading from them and giving a copy to your doctor. Sometimes, a knowledgeable nurse can provide most of the answers. Studies have been carried out on what doctors hear their patients say, and what the patients hear and recall of their physicians' statements. These studies have shown that what the doctors recall and what the patients recall are both rather faulty. You can take notes. Better still, you can audiotape the session for later listening. Meichenbaum and Turk (1987) have reviewed the literature on *adherence*, that is, how well patients carry out their doctors' instructions. Adherence or compliance is surprisingly low, and is mainly due to improper recall. The treatment for diabetes mellitus, for example, is very well-known and the regimen is conducive to leading a near-to-normal life. The regimen is not burdensome given the benefits. Yet, according to Meichenbaum and Turk, compliance by diabetics is typically less than fifty per cent. Take notes, make audiotapes, and ask for written instructions.

Some physicians provide printed hand-outs that are quite comprehensive. Often, the office nurse will explain what is in the hand-outs. The trend toward 'defensive' medicine is producing more of this kind of detailed information.

It is your choice as to your attitude towards your physician. Let me tell you a personal story. A few years ago I had to change physicians. A knowledgeable friend highly recommended a Dr. George Jones (fictitious name). He took a personal history in his office prior to the initial physical examination. I suggested that we work together on a first-name basis. "After all," I said, "if you insist on my addressing you as Doctor, then I can insist on your addressing me as Professor." George was very open to this way of working collaboratively. About one year later, we happened to be chatting about the distinctions between patient and client, and George commented that he was certain that none of the other six physicians in his group practice would be open to being called by their first name. In his office, I do not overdo the first-name thing, and I am sensitive to office protocol.

One of the things I really like about George is that I always have the sense that I have his undivided attention when I am with him. I am also certain that he will sit with me and answer all my questions, no matter how long it takes. I do not take undue advantage of his way of being with patients. The level of mutual respect and trust that we feel for each other is healing in its truest sense.

On the other hand, the most common complaint about doctors that arises in many support groups has to do with doctors not listening, or being too busy and rushed to answer questions. You can confront your doctor directly about unanswered questions and what you do not like in his behavior. Since your relationship with your doctor can have a powerful effect on the course of your disease, then be direct with him on what he does that is helpful or harmful in your interactions. For example, if hugs are important to you, then ask your doctor for a hug. Also, tell your doctors what you do like about the way they interact with you—this is a two-way relationship.

Oncology nurses and other specialty nurses are generally well-informed about all aspects of their doctor's work. They also may have more time to sit with you and explain the treatment, preparation for the treatment, side-effects, what to expect after the

Figure 5.2: But, Doc, I have some more questions … .

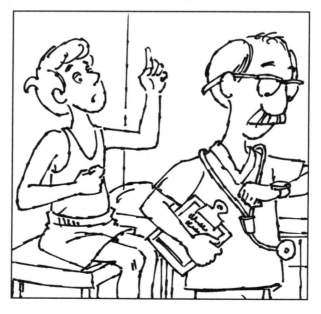

treatment, and how to care for yourself or a significant other. They too can be asked for hugs.

We all know of people who, as patients, are aggressively demanding, rude, or simply nasty. In principle, the medical establishment should treat these people no differently than a courteous or undemanding person. The aggressive patient *may* be able to influence the system and get things out of it that others cannot. But, given human nature, these pushy patients generally get short-changed by the system. This doesn't mean that you should fawn over your doctor and be a wimp. It is possible to be assertive *and* polite, demanding *and* courteous, firm *and* respectful. People respond to politeness. There is a major difference between deference or awe and respect. In all likelihood, medicine works best, both for curing and healing, when it is done cooperatively and collaboratively. Does your doctor work *on* you or *with* you? If the former, you should consider switching after sharing your feelings about how you have been treated, and giving each other the opportunity to establish a more collaborative relationship. (See the patient/oncologist statement in Appendix D.)

Remember, as a client and consumer you have choices. These choices are not just about the physician—they include treatments, tests, and facilities. Norman Cousins wrote about his heart attack (1984). A few days after the attack, he was scheduled for a stress test. Upon entering the test facility, he found it cold, mechanical, and intimidating. He canceled the test. His physician reacted with concern, and told him how important this test was for designing his treatment protocol. Cousins agreed, and told his doctor that he would take the stress test if his favorite music was played, and if some paintings (reproductions) were hung in the room. This was done and Cousins proved to be a very cooperative patient. There are many things like this that are under your control.

You have the right, perhaps even the obligation, to seek out second and third opinions. The big city in my area (Dayton) has a number of good hospitals and oncologists. Yet, sixty miles away, there is one of the major cancer hospitals and research centers in the country, the James Cancer Hospital of the Ohio State University. When a second or third opinion is necessary, clients have other options like visiting the James or Sloan-Kettering or M.D. Anderson specialty hospitals, for example. The physicians in those centers are more likely to be aware of experimental protocols, and may even be doing research in your specific type of cancer. It is also wise to seek out physicians and hospitals that specialize in a particular disease for second opinions. You can find out about such specialized centers via the web and disease-oriented hotlines.

Have your doctors communicate with each other. It is useful to have your personal physician or oncologist serve as the central person for coordinating your tests and treatments and follow-ups. Otherwise, you can get lost in the system between all of the specialists. You can also use a family member or friend as a coordinator of services.

My mother was fond of saying, "One hand washes the other." Work cooperatively with your medical helpers. If you are involved in alternative therapies, do not forget that traditional scientific Western medicine also has a lot to offer, and you should hedge your bets by availing yourself of *all* modes of help.

5.5 *Helplessness, Hopelessness, and Control*

Somewhere in their training, many medical people were cautioned about the dangers of giving false hope. There was an unspoken implication that such 'false hope' would somehow harm the recipient. After all, if a patient expects too much from a given treatment, they are then being set up for disappointment. And that it is that disappointment is presumably harmful that might lead to depression or a sense of hopelessness. So doctors are told:

- Don't promise more than you can deliver.
- Be honest and accurate and scientific in your prognoses and predictions.
- Tell the truth, no matter how devastating it may be.
- The principle of informed consent means that you have to inform patients about possible side-effects and predicted outcomes based on your experience and knowledge and the literature.

Of course, doctors do not necessarily carry out these guidelines with the coldness implied in the statements. Clients vary significantly in how much factual detail they want. Some may want it 'straight,' though most can really 'hear it all' only over time. Just as objectionable as this straight talk is the physician who glosses over the information, depriving the client of information that helps the client feel in control, and thereby manage all his resources (e.g. time, money, energy) based on the prognosis. The bulleted approach above may be mechanically and legally correct, but it is not compassionate. It ignores the folk wisdom of, "Where there is life, there is hope." This common-sense statement is the driving force for exploring alternative therapies. So, what is wrong with hope? Is there some formula that combines giving hope with informed consent?

The first devastating statement a physician may make is, "You have cancer," (or some other life-challenging disease). It is still probably true that most people who hear these words take them as a sentence of imminent death. There is also a fear that the progress of the disease necessarily involves not only pain, but unbearable pain. Is there some way to present a diagnosis of cancer that is less crushing? "The test results indicate that you have a kind of cancer that is treatable." "You are lucky that we caught this cancer at such an early stage." "Most people with this kind of cancer lead normal lives with treatment." It would be cruel to present the diagnosis in any other way if it is at all possible to speak in these hopeful ways, given the type of cancer and its stage. The lay person does not generally know that there are many different kinds of cancer, and that each one has its own typical course of development. As a patient you are entitled to this kind of information.

What if the cancer is a particularly malignant type that is fast-growing, or may have already metastasized? Can the doctor still hold out hope? The second kind of devastating statement a doctor can give is, "Your cancer is too advanced for treatment." or "We've done everything known to modern medical science. I'm sorry." These are direct no-hope statements that imply that you should immediately make out your will, tidy up your affairs, and say your goodbyes. An alternative compassionate statement might be, "I am not sure what else to do at this time. Let's continue working together. I'll keep checking the literature. We'll do whatever we can to keep you comfortable. I'll certainly help you in whatever you wish to do or try. You can always call upon me to talk or for advice. We're in this together. With your permission, I'd like to have a hospice involved in your care while I continue working with you.

Hospices provides a wide variety of services for you and your family. They can be very helpful in many ways during this transition time. You should also know that some people do graduate from hospice services. No matter what, we'll keep working together. You know, I'd like a hug now. [Caution: some patients will not want to be hugged.]"

For some people, offers to pray together are important. Since hope is such an important part of healing, hope should always be offered. No matter how adverse the circumstances, the person with the disease *always has the choice about how to respond* to what the doctor says. Feeling hopeless can have profound physical effects—so can feeling hope.

Our modern efficient medical delivery systems were typically designed for the convenience of medical personnel and their associated health management colleagues, although many things have changed and are changing with a focus on client comfort and service. There are seemingly endless forms to fill out, many of them incomprehensible. The system almost appears to be Kafka-esque in design, and is structured more like an assembly line than a healing relationship between one human being and another. Hospital and office routines can engender a sense of helplessness in the patient. This feeling of helplessness can be harmful to health, and patients need to develop empowering skills, ways of taking control over their passage through the medical system. One example of doing this was cited earlier—the way Norman Cousins approached taking a stress test. The rest of this section is devoted to ways of being in control of your medical experiences.

a. *Medical Records*. What is written about you is written about *you*, and you have the right to both read and obtain copies of all of your medical records. Although there may be things written in your records that you do not understand, they are still yours. You can always ask some knowledgeable person, perhaps a medical reference librarian, to 'translate.' Your doctor and his nurse should be willing to explain what is in your records. You can also request that copies of records (or the records themselves) be sent to another physician or clinic. Be persistent when you encounter resistance obtaining or reviewing your medical records.

Figure 5.3: Reading your own medical records.

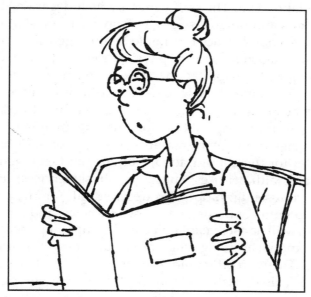

b. *Ombudsman.* Almost all hospitals now have an ombudsman or patient representative/advocate on their staff. You can use these people to represent your interests with the hospital. They can expedite procedures and obtain answers quickly. They are paid to be *your* advocate within the system, and their knowledge of procedure and protocol works for you. A member of your family or a friend can sometimes serve the same function. (They may need to have your written authorization.)

c. *Pastoral Staff.* Most hospitals employ, or have available, pastoral staff (hospital chaplains) to help patients with religious and spiritual concerns. The chaplain can also serve as an advocate, and as someone with 'inside' information on the workings of a hospital. They will pray with you and spend time with you and listen to you. Chaplains generally have links with community resources such as support groups, social aid, and legal aid. The medical social services department is also a good source for information and community resources. You do not need to be religious yourself, or of the denomination of the chaplain, to request his services. Of course, you can also ask your own minister or pastor or rabbi to visit.

d. *Hospital Social Services Department*. These services are free if you are a hospital patient. The staff generally includes trained medical social workers and nurse discharge planners. These staff members will serve as your contact for: home health agencies (care in the home from a registered nurse, physical therapist, aide, or home-maker); inpatient rehabilitation services; extended care facilities such as nursing homes; hospice care services; adult day centers; and hospital-to-hospital transfers. They are also a link to community services such as: transportation for ongoing treatments such as dialysis or chemotherapy or radiation therapy; prescription assist-ance; shelter for the abused; food, clothing, and emergency hous-ing; mental health services; substance abuse services; individual and group counseling; support groups; referrals for financial assist-ance to help with continuing care resource costs; and family coun-seling. They will assist in explaining and completing the 'advanced directives' known as living wills and durable power of attorney for health care. They can offer guidance on financial matters relating to health care. This department can assist in obtaining your doctor-approved durable medical equipment such as walkers, wheel-chairs, and hospital beds. The nurse discharge planner will explain after-hospital medication and care, as this may be particularly important. As a hospital patient, you should avail yourself of these free services, and also of the community health services they can connect you to.

e. *Clothing and Room Decor*. The clothing issued to patients in hos-pitals is designed for the convenience of the staff. By all means, bring your own pajamas or nightgowns, bathrobe, and slippers. Leisure clothing like sweat suits or work-out clothes may also be worn. Be comfortable in your own familiar clothing. You can add your own pillow, and cover your bed with your own bedspread, quilt, or afghan.

Personalize the decor of your room. An artist friend could not stand the institutional art in her room and covered the picture with a favorite colorful shawl. You could also hang (with permission) per-sonal art work, but check this out before bringing in the art work. Many hospitals have a lending library of art work.

It appears to be the case that patients in rooms with views of sky and greenery do better than those in interior rooms with no views,

Figure 5.4: Decorating your hospital room!

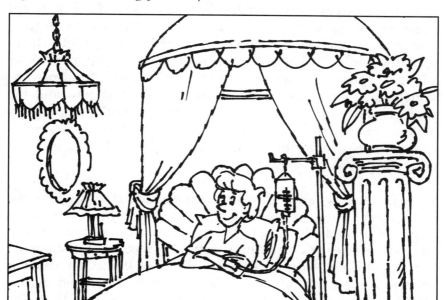

or views of other buildings. At the minimum, you have contact with the weather. Visual vistas do something for inner peace. Ask to get a room with a view of the outside world, preferably one that looks out on greenery.

It is not only children who are comforted by stuffed toy animals. For some reason, having a special stuffed animal or other toy can be comforting. Many nursing homes, for example, encourage the practice of residents having dolls or stuffed animals. There are hospitals that permit visits of pets, or have their own visiting pet program.

You never know how much of your physical environment is under your control until you test the system. If the first response is "No," being insistent may get results.

f. *Examinations*. You can refuse to be examined or to take a particular test. You may be able to modify the conditions of the test, as Norman Cousins did. Some examination conditions may be under your control. Here are four stories that are good examples.

The following story was told to me by a mutual friend of Harriet's. She was hospitalized with an abdominal problem. One morning, the chief resident was making rounds, followed by his gaggle of students. When he got to Harriet's bed, he consulted her chart and began to discuss her 'case.' He was interrupted by a loud "Ahem" from Harriet. He made his first eye contact with Harriet, whereupon she said, "Did I give you permission to talk about me?" After a longish pause the chief resident said, "May I have your permission to talk about your case?" Harriet looked at him and the students and simply said, "No." The doctor, dutifully followed by his students, had to move on. Harriet was not a 'case' or a 'possible gall bladder.' Examinations and discussions of your disease need your permission.

There is a story of an artist who was hospitalized for a while. She had a friend bring an easel, a large pad of newsprint, and a collection of colored felt-tipped pens. This woman would not let anyone examine her or do anything in the room without first paying her 'fee' of doing a drawing. This worked well until a particular resident came to examine her. She explained the procedure. He said that he didn't have the time and that he couldn't draw. She said, "No examination." They were log-jammed until she said, "Do you have any money?" At first he was non-plussed, then he looked in his pockets. "I have thirty-five cents." She said, "That's enough. Put the money on my tray and you can examine me." He did.

Bernie Siegel tells the following story which he found in a longer version in the *Journal of the American Medical Association*:

> A nineteen year old boy was in the hospital to die and the crazy routine made no sense when you considered what he was there for. He had a sign over his bed which read, "Interns shot on sight," and used a water gun to release his anger without hurting anyone. The staff never took the gun away, and when he died it was given by the boy's mother to an intern who befriended him. This intern gave the gun to an eight year old to empower him when he was being worked over for leukemia.

This is K'Anna Burton's surgery story (2000, printed with her permission):

> Cancer came to my door recently. It was unexpected. There may be an "epidemic" of it out there somewhere, but a melanoma in my left

ear? Why me? Why in my left ear? There are always more questions than answers. I may have more questions than usual since I am an adjunct professor in the Holistic Health Care program at Western Michigan University (Kalamazoo). I am also a massage and body work therapist.

Unfortunately, my dermatologist surgeon was straight protocol. He was impatient with my questions and my holistic approach to health and healing. Due to a number of circumstances—the most important was his reputation as a skilled surgeon—I nevertheless chose to keep him as my doctor. Still, somehow, I wanted to shift his internal personal energies in ways that would best enhance my healing and well-being. Any surgery is scary, and cancer surgery is scarier. What to do?

Since talking with the surgeon directly was not a real choice, I decided to send him a greeting card. In the card I wrote, "I want to thank you for the time you spent with me and my questions. I look forward to your best work in my upcoming surgery, and am comforted to be in such competent hands. Thank you."

The morning of my surgery arrived. Somehow, his personality seemed softer, and he was more personally concerned. The surgery went very well. A few weeks later I sent him another card, this time expressing my genuine feelings of thanks.

This may be a simple thing, yet both cards conveyed my heart-felt feelings, and both were "heard" by this surgeon. Although he appeared to be engrossed in the mechanics of identifying and removing cancers, the cards served as a reminder of the profound effect that his human-ness, and his gentler personality, could have on his patients in their healing process. We can all benefit from these "simple" reminders. For me the good feelings that came from just taking charge of this aspect of my healing journey have allowed me to share this story with many others. And, these sharings have been very well received!

It is a common complaint, almost a cliché, that hospital food is awful. The menus may be nutritionally correct for you at that time, but there is a large leeway in diets. There is no sense to a 'correct' meal if you find it unpalatable and do not eat it, or selectively eat a portion. Talk to the food staff about your likes and dislikes. Friends and relatives can bring in hot dishes you like. If you have trouble feeding yourself, then a friend or relative may (or may not!—your choice) make this easier. Many hospice facilities have kitchens so you can prepare your own food or have someone prepare a favorite food on the spot. Some even have smoking rooms for those patients who are smokers—a level of compassion and consideration that is commendable. In one hospice, all patient rooms look out on a green area with a bird feeder. Ducks from a nearby pond walk that area. Most hospices have an armchair in the room that is convertible to a single bed, and a separate toilet and shower facility for family. All of this is thoughtful and helpful.

There are lots of ways to empower yourself. For example, if there is a particular technician or nurse who makes you feel uncomfortable, or whom you dislike for *any* reason, you can request that a different person work with you. There is no reason to tolerate a brusque or rude technician in the radiation facility, for example. Bernie Siegel has commented that patients that staff complain about as being uncooperative, or even too demanding, appear to be the survivors. About these complaints he has written (private communication, 2000), "What I am talking about is survival and immune competent behavior. There are patterns in long-term survivors which doctors don't learn about or teach unless they learn from their own illness." On the other hand, the overly compliant and docile patients appear not to survive as well. Remember, again, that there are great differences between being abusively demanding, politely assertive, and passively compliant. For example, Cindy always got what she wanted and needed from medical personnel because she was so undemandingly loving that the staff just wanted to be in her presence, even hang out in her room when they had a spare minute or two. Her special healer was a personal angel. In a way she was an angel herself. One needs to be cautious here, since it is certainly not the case that being true to yourself, if that means being gentle and non-assertive, for example, hastens death—there are many ways to get your needs met, assertiveness is just one.

5.6 *'Mechanical' Matters, Wills, etc.*

By 'mechanical' matters, I mean all of those practical considerations that need to be attended to with some urgency by people who have life-challenging diseases and their families. Of course, prudence dictates that many of these matters should be taken care of when you are well and there is no urgency. They are separately discussed in what follows.

a. *Wills*. A legally binding will gives directions about the disposition of your worldly possessions after death. Most couples will everything to the survivor, with further provisions for both dying at the same time or within a short time of each other. It is generally best to consult a lawyer for writing a complex will. If your estate is simple, there are clever computer programs available at nominal cost that will help you write your will, with specific provisions to make it legal within your state (in the U.S.). You must also comply with provisions for notarizing or witnesses. Copies of your will can be deposited with your bank, your lawyer, your children, friends, and the designated executor of your will. The will can be sealed or open.

When nearing the end of life, some choose to give themselves the pleasure of giving away cherished items to children, grandchildren, and friends. There's a way now to donate assets to a charitable organization that lets you, for example, keep the dividends of stocks until your death, when the assets belong to the charity. Estate planning is important, period. There are specialists who can help you with this for a fee.

b. *The Living Will*. The living will is your way to give instructions to your family and to your medical team about your medical care if you become incapacitated and can't directly convey your wishes. The living will specifies just what care and interventions you are willing to have in the last stages of your life. For example, you can specify that no extraordinary measures or resuscitation methods be used. Living wills need to be properly executed and witnessed and filed with relevant people, according to the laws of your state. For your information, a sample living will (valid in Ohio) is included as Appendix E. At the end is an example of a completed living will. These choices need to be discussed with your spouse, family, doctor, minister, or friends. A living will is a *personal* statement. (*Christian Affirmation of Life* is in Appendix F and *The Christian Living Will* is in Appendix G.)

The written contract you sign when you are eligible for hospice care (usually a prognosis of six months or less for life) contains agreements similar to a living will. This contract should be carefully studied. You typically agree that no extraordinary measures will be used to prolong life. Since 'extraordinary measures' are open to interpretation, you need to be as specific as possible in this area. Again, it is well to execute a living will when you are in good health. It is always possible to change a living will as your circumstances change.

c. *Durable Power of Attorney for Health Care.* A power of attorney gives another person or an institution the legal authority to represent your interests. It can designate *specific limited* powers, for example, money, assets, guardianship, etc. The *durable power of attorney for health care* document comes into force by a conscious act if you are sentient and can communicate, or automatically if you can no longer make decisions for yourself (a court may be involved in such a decision). Among other matters, it empowers your executor to make decisions about medical treatment on your behalf. These instructions need to be legally written and witnessed and filed. Different states have different requirements. For your information, a sample durable power of attorney for health care (valid in Ohio) is included as Appendix H.

You also need to be aware that some doctors, nurses, and hospitals may not be willing to honor your choices in a living will or of your executor for a durable power of attorney for health care. If not, they are required to say so, and to give you other options for service. Always check in advance with your personal physician and any specialists whose services you anticipate using. Also check on the policies of your area hospitals. All these medical people and institutions should give you clear and easily understandable responses. You can change doctors and specify particular hospitals. This is one reason to execute these documents in advance.

d. *Medical Insurance.* The one area that seems to get people hotter under the collar than any other is medical insurance. There are a variety of coverages: Medicaid, Medicare, personally paid-for private plans, supplemental plans, and employer-contracted plans. However, some individuals fall through the cracks in the system because they have no medical coverage whatsoever. With the prevalence of managed care, despite all of the fine print and PR flummery, it is frequently difficult to know what is covered by a particular plan, and to what extent. The paper work for an outpatient procedure or an office visit can continue for months and months before it is resolved. You need to be persistent, keep all paper records, and document each step. There are 800 numbers to call for almost everything. Once you have persisted through the 'if this, press that,' you may get some answers and some satisfaction.

A major difficulty with managed care arises if there is a conflict between what your doctor recommends for your care and what the system permits. For example, an oncologist recommended a particular course of chemotherapy for a client whose insurance company refused to authorize the treatment. This refusal was despite the doctor's recommendation and the citation of literature studies indicating that this course of treatment was 25 to 35 per cent effective for his cancer. The client died before all of the channels within the insurance company had been exhausted. One recourse that some insured people take when a particular treatment has been denied is to seek legal counsel and to sue the insurance company. Legal maneuvers take time and effort and energy and money that might otherwise be spent on yourself and your healing. If it is too draining for you to pursue these matters relating to medical insurance, you need to recruit an advocate from family or friends. The old advice of 'sue the bastards' might be another recourse.

The National Coalition for Cancer Survivorship (NCCS) will send a free booklet entitled *What Cancer Survivors Need to Know About Health Insurance*, which is also applicable to other diseases (877-622-7937). NCCS will also send a useful free audio tape on finding ways to pay for care.

e. *Financial Matters*. A will meets legal requirements for disposing of your estate after you die. But the complexity of inheritance laws and probating a will means that you need to do estate planning well before you die. There are books and computer programs and financial advisers to help you in these matters. One person took care of all the details in his estate, and each of his children has a loose-leaf binder with all of the information. In fact, he has already made his funeral arrangements and paid for them. Even though we may feel immortal as a teenager, no one gets out of this world alive! Plan accordingly. There are ways to minimize inheritance taxes and shorten probate. It is not considerate to dump this on your children if your health allows you to do this planning yourself.

f. *End-of-Life Care Plan.* Meyer and Kaplan (1998) have written thoughtfully about the necessity of an end-of-life care plan that incorporates some of the materials in this section. Since their comments are so useful, they are quoted here.

> To ensure that a person's end-of-life wishes are honored and their personal values respected, a reasonably complete End-of-Life Care Plan is essential. The major purpose of an End-of-Life Care Plan is to set goals for medical treatment and for social, emotional, and spiritual supports in all stages of a person's care from the time they face serious illness or decline until their death. The plan also must include a process for reviewing and evaluating the goals from time to time. Ideally, the patient, the patient's loved ones, and the health care team construct a Care Plan together. If the patient cannot participate in the planning, the designated health care agent or other appropriate surrogates should be involved. Although the physician recommends and prescribes medical care elements of the plan, the wishes and personal values of the patient should guide these elements as well. In addition to addressing the types of desirable medical treatments, the plan should take into account such things as the patient's spiritual values and beliefs, family concerns, where the patient would like to die, concerns about pain and suffering, and financial considerations. An End-of-Life Care Plan should be in place any time a person faces significant life changes or health care problems that are likely to result in decline and perhaps death. Finally, the planning process should involve a discussion of advance directives and the completion of documents.

Under the heading of *Who should suggest creating a care plan?* Meyer and Kaplan write:

> Ideally, the physician should raise the question of care planning as part of a discussion in which questions or treatment alternatives are raised. But, often, for one reason or another, the health care team does not initiate planning. It is up to each of us, as patient or patient's advocate, to raise planning questions with the health care team.... Our health care system is so complex that it is unwise to assume that others will initiate discussions about end-of-life care planning.

Finally, they end up with seven parts of working with a care plan that includes the Choice in Dying 800 telephone number:

- Focus on the patient's personal goals for care. Review existing advanced directives or complete new ones. Be certain that the patient's goals are clearly identified.
- Measure any recommended medical treatments or actions against the patient's goals for end-of-life care.
- Ask questions about treatments. Ask about other options such as palliative care or hospice care, which are focused on the patient's comfort.
- Be persistent in seeking information.
- Revisit the plan periodically.
- Try to avoid creating adversarial relationships. The goal is to create a partnership between the medical professionals and the patient, or the patient's surrogate, for the benefit of the patient.
- If you cannot establish a successful working relationship or if you do not feel the medical team is responsive to your concerns, seek other help. You can request a second opinion, talk to a patient representative or an administrator, or call Choice in Dying (800-989-9455) for other suggestions.

g. *Suicide and Euthanasia.* A Chicago resident, Charles, had cancer and was in the last stages of his life. There was a surprise gathering of Charles' friends at a cook-out for him. As Charles entered the room, he exclaimed, "Aha, the Last Supper!" A man with a sense of humor and much spirit. After two days, he needed life support to breathe. A week after the 'last supper,' and with his family about him, Charles asked his doctor to pull the plug. The doctor did. Was this suicide? Euthanasia? Illegal? Moral? Murder? Although there are legal constraints and legal definitions that differ widely, the answers to these serious questions are ultimately personal. Some family members and friends make private agreements about various life contingencies. It is wise to think about these issues and the legal and moral and religious implications before circumstances force such considerations upon you.

The group Aging With Dignity (P.O. Box 1661, Tallahassee, FL 32302-1661; 850-681-2010) has prepared an easy-to-understand booklet (just a few pages) that makes it easier "to let your doctor, family, and friends know how you want to be treated," if you become seriously ill and cannot tell them. This booklet addresses:

My wish for:

1. The person I want to make care decisions for me when I can't.
2. The kind of medical treatment I want or don't want.
3. How comfortable I want to be.
4. How I want people to treat me.
5. What I want my loved ones to know.

The *Five Wishes* are obtainable for $5.00 per copy from Aging With Dignity (address above). They also sell a helpful video.

Do you have a right to die with dignity? Are all parts of the process under your control? Can you guarantee no harm to others if you make such a choice? There is a vast literature on this subject now, and much debate. There are also groups like the Hemlock Society (P.O. Box 101810, Denver, CO 80250-1810; 800-247-7421) that provide information about these things. For a person with a life-challenging disease and his family, these questions are no longer theoretical. Consider them with care and concern.

5.7 Communicating with Others— Relationships

If you do have cancer or some other serious disease, how do you communicate? How much do you share about your treatment? Your feelings? Your fears? Your concerns? With whom do you share and when? All of the time? Rarely? Only when they ask?

All relationships seem to change once you've been diagnosed with a life-challenging disease. It is not unknown, cruel as it may appear, for the healthy wife or husband to seek a divorce. This decision may be opportunistic, financially the only recourse, or it may be that he or she just does not know how to cope with such a catastrophic event in their partner's life. Some gay partners remain together when one is diagnosed with AIDS, others separate, some flee. A wedding service may include the words, "In sickness and in health," and, "Till death do us part," but these solemn vows may not survive events like an auto accident that causes quadriplegia. How well do you (and can you) know your life partner? Relationships evolve through time and circumstance, but life-challenging and debilitating diseases can and do wreak havoc on relationships. Who do you turn to? What can you do? (The workbook in Section 4.3 is a private way to communicate with yourself and a private outlet for your feelings.)

Figure 5.5: Really sharing your feelings.

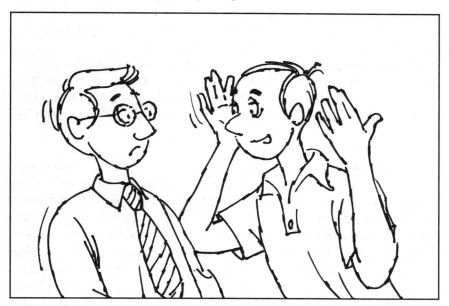

Since medicine is a doctor's *chosen* profession, you can presumably say anything to your doctors, and also ask them anything. Some aspects relating to this were discussed above. Yet, you will find many doctors who are uncomfortable when you want to share personal feelings, when you become emotional, or when you show signs of 'hysteria' or depression. If you can't communicate with your doctor, then a counselor, psychotherapist, social worker or minister may be your next choice. Only physicians and/or psychiatrists can prescribe medication. Some psychoactive drugs can be quite helpful to get you over the initial shock and distress of a diagnosis. Used wisely, a relaxant or sleeping pills can get you to the point where you are thinking more clearly and are ready to take charge of your life and make your own choices. Some people avoid prescription drugs on principle, but when taken for a specific purpose and in a time-limited way, they can be most beneficial in a tough spot. By all means get the effects and side-effects explained to you.

It is common with people who have a life-challenging disease to notice that some friends no longer call, and that some relatives become remote. On an overt level, being in the presence of someone who has cancer or AIDS, for example, is a forceful reminder of mortality. People who can't handle that thought in themselves, or who can't acknowledge the mortality of someone they love, cut themselves off to deny the idea of death. You will most likely experience the shock of losing some close friends and relatives, *and* the surprise of new supportive relationships. You can give short shrift to the morbidly curious, those strange people who want to know all of the 'details.' Your life is none of their business. One woman who grew tired of well-meaning queries about her health simply states, "I'm fine; there are just some parts of me that are not."

You will need to calibrate relationships in terms of your own needs. You can say in a support group things you could never say to your family, for example. There may be one friend you can 'dump' on in the sense of falling apart, crying, and giving voice to your deepest fears. The networking and friendships that develop within support groups are very helpful, but you need to be assertive about using this resource. They are *your* people, and you can be comfortable with them since they have been through or are going through the same experiences as you. There is an instant rapport with sisters who have had lumpectomies, with brothers who have had radical prostatectomies, and anyone who has lived through a series of radiation treatments. You become part of another culture with all of its rites, rituals, ceremonies, and secret words.

The National Coalition for Cancer Survivorship (NCCS) provides two useful audio programs free of charge. They are: *Cancer Survival Toolbox* and *Topics for Older Persons*. Contact 877-622-7937 or visit their website: www.cansearch.org.

5.8 Support Networks

A single person with cancer or some other serious disease can be quickly overwhelmed by the demands made of him and his family. If you are employed, there are all the arrangements that have to be made about time off, insurance, etc. If you are a homemaker, your partner may end up with employment concerns. The family's life gets disrupted; new routines need to be established. The person who is ill may need some help with home care depending on where he is in his treatment and the progress of the disease. How do you manage your changed life? One way to do this is to set up a support network. There are similarities and differences as to how this is done depending on whether you are single or married.

If you are single, call a meeting of concerned friends to set up your support network. The organization of this meeting may best be done by a friend who has the time and is willing to serve as your support network coordinator. Before the meeting, prepare a list of *specific* things that you need from your supporters. This list may include some or all of the following items:

(1) *Who will be the coordinator*? This service may be performed in rotation by several people.
(2) *Transportation*. Who will drive you to your different appointments when you cannot do this by yourself?
(3) *Food*. Who will buy food for you? Who will prepare meals? Who washes the dishes? Meals can be brought in, or you may go to that person's house.
(4) *Cleaning*. Who will make arrangements for cleaning your house and coordinate volunteers to do this?
(5) *Laundry*. Who will handle the laundry?
(6) *Garden and Yard*. If you live in a house with a garden and/or yard, who will take care of this, e.g., mow the lawn, rake the leaves, and weed?
(7) *House/Apartment Maintenance*. Who will be available to fix things that need repair, or to find service people, or to move furniture?
(8) *Children*. If you have children living at home, who will care for them? Baby-sit when you are away? Take them to and from school? Feed them? See to their needs? Play with them? Help them study? Arrange to transport them to activities? Arrange time with their friends?
(9) *Financial*. Do you need assistance financially to pay for your treatments? Do you need financial advice? Can someone raise money for you or assist with obtaining financial help?
(10) *Legal*. Do you need help with a will or a living will or a durable power of attorney for health care or other legal matters?

(11) *Medical Insurance.* Do you need someone to check your coverage and to be your representative/advisor with your medical insurance provider?

(12) *Hospitals.* Who will help you deal with your hospital(s) and their paperwork and bills and appointments?

(13) *Medical Care.* Do you have *one* doctor who is in overall charge of your treatment? Ideally, all medical services and reports should be channeled through this one physician. You may also need a lay person who helps with communicating with doctors, and who is willing to research options for medical care.

(14) *Counseling.* Do you have a trusted mental health worker in whom you can confide and to whom you can divulge your innermost feelings?

(15) *Information.* Can one person or a team help with obtaining, organizing, and reviewing relevant information?

(16) *Fun.* Do not forget to party, to socialize, to have fun, to go out—someone may be able to coordinate fun activities.

Remember one of Rabbi Hillel's questions: "If you are not for yourself, who will be?"

Figure 5.6: Assigning tasks to your support network.

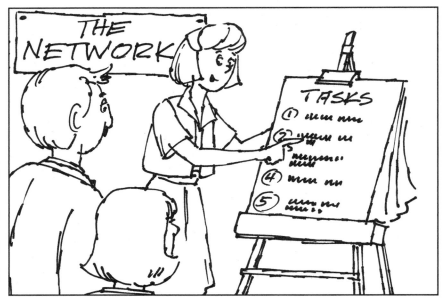

Let's look at this again. Most of us were brought up to be selfless, to think of the other person first, to do good deeds. But in this world, by and large, you will not get things if you do not directly ask for them. Wishing and dreaming and praying may work, but asking is better. The worst thing than can happen is that you encounter a "No." Ask again. Ask someone else. In this sense, you need to be somewhat selfish to get your needs met. This is not only okay, it is in effect demanded by the circumstances. There is an adage, "Ask nicely." So, ask nicely, but ask!

For a person with a family, a family member may serve as the convener and organizer of your support network. This network would include both family and friends. You still need to do the homework of preparing a specific list of needs. It may be harder to be 'selfish' within the family—it still needs to be done to get needs met.

You may be part of a religious or social group that already has mechanisms in place to establish a support network for you. Contact them and use them. There are professional helping services available that can provide most of what you need. Some charge, and some do not. You may need to hire a cleaning person or a private duty nurse.

If you become part of a hospice program, they have professional staff who care for your needs in many categories. In areas where they do not directly provide a service you need, their social worker can direct you to relevant resources.

You do not have to go through this alone—reach out and someone will take your hand.

5.9 *Counseling and Psychotherapy*

When you're stuck and emotionally up against a wall, you can consider going to a counselor or psychotherapist for emotional support and understanding. He will help you find ways of coping with your situation. This *may* be a good time to work through unfinished business from the past. The choice is yours. If the disease is creating difficulties in relationships with your spouse, your family, with significant others, or at work, then therapy can be helpful. There are therapists who specialize in working with couples, with families, and with those who have life-challenging diseases. It is important to get a good match. If the therapist is not helpful, find another one. There are also ministers who specialize in this kind of work (but do not expect all to be prepared for this). If you think that medication will be helpful, then approach your doctor or a psychiatrist. "If I am not for myself, … "

Figure 5.7: Praying with a friend.

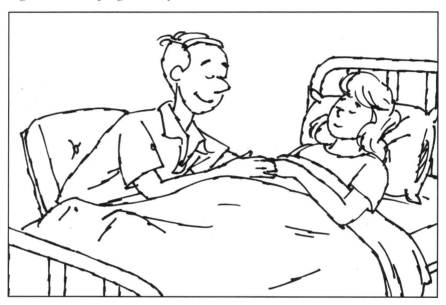

5.10 Prayer and Religious Support

There are a number of interesting studies (see Dossey, 1991, 1993, 1996, 1997 for details on the usefulness of prayer) indicating the power of prayer in healing. This is prayer by the affected person, his family, his church, and by groups who can be unknown to you. If praying is important to you, then by all means pray, and make arrangements for others to pray for and with you. Prayer allows us to say things aloud that we may be uncomfortable saying in a regular conversation.

Some people benefit mightily from religious retreats, personal support from their minister, and support from their church, others do not. One woman would no longer let her minister visit, since he was so obviously uncomfortable in her presence—this was painful to her. Again, you need to calibrate this kind of support to find out what is helpful to you.

Figure 5.8: Helping another hospital patient.

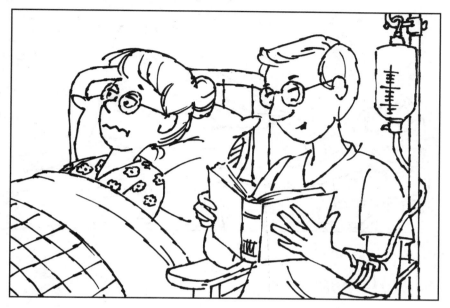

5.11 Helping Others

Even though you may be distressed, uncomfortable, and in pain, there may still be ways in which you can help others. Just like you cannot touch without being touched, you can't help others without being helped yourself. At the minimum, you are not giving up, giving in, or being helpless. There are still useful things you can do. If you are in a hospital, there may be fellow patients who are less mobile than you are. Can you visit with them, read to them, listen to them? If you are bed-ridden, then perforce you are a captive audience to whoever visits you. Can you listen and respond in ways that are helpful to your visitors, the nurses, the staff, your doctors? No matter the circumstances, there are always choices. You can decide to be a passive or an active participant. Remember, the best gift you can give is being receptive to gifts, letting or *asking* others to do things for you. If you are mobile, then there are many ways you can help others. The more you help, the more you are helped.

Figure 5.9: Relaxing with a therapeutic massage.

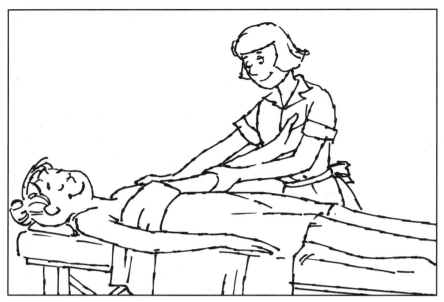

5.12 *Massage*

One of life's great joys can be a full-body massage, preferably for 45 to 60 minutes. A good masseur is knowledgeable about all sorts of bodily aches and pains and knows just where to press or smooth to ease discomforts and release muscle strains. Some massage therapists are not confident about massaging people who have cancer. Of course, you need to be careful where you are massaged, and just how much pressure is used. With care and caution, massage can do wonders for people who have life-challenging diseases. Check it out. The March/April 2000 issue of *Massage* has three articles on massage with cancer patients (Williams, 2000; Kirby, 2000; Mac-Donald, 2000). These articles present guidelines for the massage therapist as well as many examples of how massage can be beneficial. According to the authors, massage can be a positive part of most treatment regimens.

You should also be aware that there are many schools of massage—some are quite gentle, while others may use a great deal of pressure. Shiatsu, for example, uses much pressure on particular acupressure points. This pressure can be adjusted for individual needs. Some facilities have their own massage people. Some hospitals permit non-staff practitioners to do massage on their premises. Again, don't be afraid to ask.

5.13 Information Sources

When people find out you have cancer or other serious diseases, they all want to give you advice and information. "Have you tried this?" "Have you read that?" "Have you consulted with?" "My brother/mother/uncle had the same thing and they...." How much information do you want and need?

The desire for information is culturally based. In Japan, for example, it is considered proper to tell a cancer patient essentially nothing about his condition and treatment. Euphemisms are frequently used like, "You have extreme stomach distress," rather than saying outright, "You have pancreatic cancer." Within the U.S. we have come a long way from the time when the word 'cancer' was only whispered, or not said out loud at all. Some people want all

Figure 5.10: Checking the Internet for information.

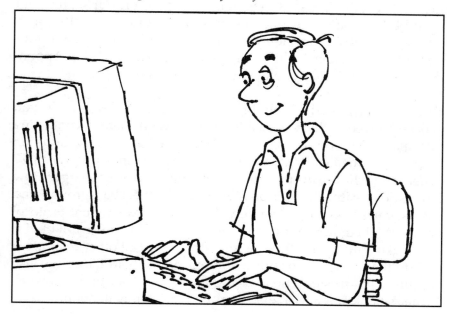

the information they can possibly get about their disease and its treatment, including technical information. Others wish to eschew information, do not want to participate in their treatment, and turn over all decisions to their doctors and/or family. For some people, hugs and information are wonderful, but others do not like being hugged or want information. Their wishes in this regard must be respected.

If you do desire information, it is readily available from a variety of sources. There is so much information available that you may not have the time or energy to explore it, let alone to study and evaluate it. You can ask your partner or a friend to take over the role of screening available information and provide you with a limited amount of material. The Worldwide Web or Internet is now the primary source of information on the disease itself and treatment options. Some good sources for cancer are the National Cancer Institute of the NIH, Medline, the American Cancer Society, and the National Center for Complementary and Alternative Medicine (NCCAM) of the NIH. There are websites for many specific diseases (kidney, lung, emphysema, AIDS, amyotrophic lateral sclerosis, etc.), which can be accessed either by the disease name or an organization for that disease. A friend who is adept at searching the Web can be of great help. So can medical school librarians, hospital reference librarians, and your local library staff. Your doctors and their staff can usually direct you to sources *and* provide you with relevant materials. For your guidance, a number of the principal websites are listed in Appendix B along with many relevant phone numbers.

Once you have studied the information, what then? How do you choose between which source to believe when there is conflicting information? If you decide to try alternative therapies (in addition to standard medical treatment), which one or ones do you pick? Where and who are the providers? How much do they charge? How long is the treatment? Is it possible to check their background and success rates? Do they accurately describe their treatment protocol or shield it behind proprietary claims? Is their literature full of glittering generalities? Do they insist that you stop all other treatments and do theirs alone? Consult with your doctor before leaping; also consult with trusted friends. For alternative cancer treatments, Lerner's book (1996) is a good starting place for evaluation.

5.14 Controlling Medication

Drugs, herbs, and other natural substances have been used for thousands of years to ease suffering and to treat diseases. Some were effective and some were not. Until about the 1950s, there were no controlled studies or real quality control on medications. Perhaps that is why it is said that until the 1950s, the history of medicine was in fact the history of the placebo effect. With the advents of regulatory agencies like the Food and Drug Administration (FDA) and double-blind studies of drugs, we are on a safer and more sound basis with respect to medications. You may be aware that some medications work better in combination, some do not, and some may even have antagonistic effects on each other. Are we an over-medicated society? Perhaps. In this section some precautions you can take are discussed.

First, have your doctor and/or his nurse explain the purpose of the medication, the dosage and regimen, the predicted useful effects, and the potential side-effects. If an information leaflet does not come with your medication, ask your pharmacist for one. The Web is also an excellent source of information on medication (see Appendix B). Check the PDR (*Physicians' Desk Reference*) for the drug you are taking—your local library should have a copy in its reference section. Ask the doctor or pharmacist about potential difficulties with taking *other* drugs, even non-prescription over-the-counter drugs, at the same time. Do you take the drug before eating? With food? After a meal? When and with what time lapses? Should you increase your intake of fluid, and to what extent? Should you avoid or restrict alcoholic beverages? Are there special foods you should take with the drug? It is usually a good idea, for example, to eat a small container of yogurt each day you are on an antibiotic to repopulate your large colon with 'good' bacteria. (*Caution*—some drugs are inactivated by dairy products.)

If you are on multiple medications, make a list of all of the drugs that you take, their dosage, when and how you take them, and note the color and shape of the drug (they are all distinctive). This is especially important if you are hospitalized and drugs are administered by the nurses. Knowing the color and shape, for instance, can help you know at a glance if you are getting the correct medication. Keep a list by your bedside. It is useful to review your list of medications periodically with your doctor. He may have forgotten some of the prescriptions—some may no longer be needed, some may have been prescribed by other physicians, some may work inappropriately with others. You may even need to consult a specialist on medication.

Figure 5.11: Which pill do I take now?

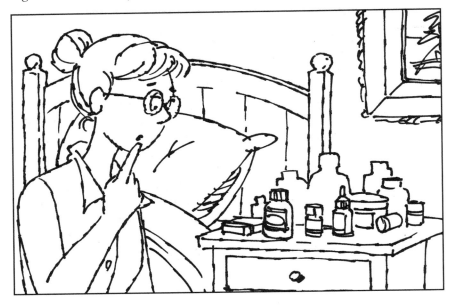

Above all, be sensitive to your own bodily reactions to a given drug. Common adverse side-effects are: nausea, diarrhea, constipation, dizziness, rashes, and dry mouth. Immediately consult your doctor about these side-effects and whether you should stop the medication or alter the dosage or switch to an alternative one. Since some medical insurance plans restrict the brand of the drug doctors may prescribe, or insist on generic drugs, you need to be sensitive to the source of the drug. In principle, generic drugs should have the same beneficial effects and side-effects of name-brand drugs, but differences have been noted. We all react to drugs differently. The doctor prescribes a 'standard' dose for your age, weight, and condition. But, some people require significantly different doses—higher *or* lower—than the standard amount. You and your doctor may need to calibrate the dosage.

Modern drugs are often amazingly effective. They can also cause harmful reactions, as in *adverse drug reactions* (ADR). The paper by

Lazarou, Pomeranz, and Covey (1998) in the respected *Journal of the American Medical Association* points out the enormous number of ADRs the researchers found in a study of the literature. They looked solely at hospital ADRs. There are even ADR-caused fatalities. You need to be very alert about the medications given to you in hospitals in particular, but also in general. Remember, you can refuse to take any medication or to participate in any treatment.

Needy Meds (334-662-0023; www.needymeds.com) is a clearing ghouse for information about obtaining medications from pharmaceutical manufacturers' assistance programs. There is no charge for this service. The Pharmaceutical Research and Manufacturers Association of America provides *The Directory of Prescription Drug Patient Assistance Programs* (1100 15th Street NW, Washington, DC 2005; www.phrma.org).

5.15 Pain Management

Western medicine has come a long way from the time when doctors were afraid to give too much pain medication because they feared their patients would become addicted. (Certainly, morphine, the preferred drug for controlling severe pain, is addictive.) The practice of pain control has changed due to two considerations. First, it makes no sense to worry about addiction for cancer or other patients in their last days, weeks, or even months. For the people who have 'graduated' from a hospice program, the problem of beating the addiction appears to be small with respect to the problems concerning re-entering the world of people with normal life expectancies. The second factor is that health care workers who work with life-challenging diseases and, particularly, hospice staff, now know a great deal more about the control of pain, and have better devices for controlling the delivery of pain medication. Many hospitals have pain clinics that specialize in the control of all kinds of pain. These clinics are staffed by a variety of professionals including medical doctors, nurses, psychiatrists, psychologists, hypnotists, and social workers.

There is now no reason to be uncomfortable or in severe pain for any significant length of time. Melzack (1990), a leading pain research scientist, recommends that it is better to give pain medication on a regular timed basis, than on demand. This is because on-demand dosing can lead to a see-saw, up-and-down, effect on comfort. The goal is to keep the patient as comfortable *and* as sentient as possible. This is best done by administering lower doses, but sufficient for sustained comfort, by slow-release pills, patches or implants, metering pumps, or a regularly timed delivery. These approaches minimize the peaks of pain and the almost comatose valleys between. The metering pumps also have an override to help control break-through pain by self-administering an extra controlled dose. Since you are the only judge of your comfort level, you need to be assertive to get what you want. People respond differently to the same dosage, and needs change with time. Ask and you shall be succored.

One of the most feared consequences of cancer is the severe pain that comes with *some* cancers, particularly in the last stages. All cancers are different, and many do not involve major pain or disability. Although cancer is specifically mentioned here, there are many other diseases where pain control is important and the ideas in this section are relevant. Remember Frankl's advice—we may not be able to control what happens to us, but we always have the choice of *how* we respond. Being held by someone you love may be the medication of choice.

5.16 Nutrition

Nutrition appears to be high on everyone's list of needed lifestyle changes when they are confronted by a life-challenging disease. Unfortunately, there appears to be little consensus about the best diet for any given condition, except, perhaps, for diabetes mellitus. (In the last stages of life, diet is a small issue.) There are major dietary regimens like macrobiotics and vegetarian (which has many variations). Book after book has been published lauding the virtues of some particular diet that the author is convinced got rid of his cancer or cured lupus, for example. The truth of the matter is that each and every one of these special diets has probably helped someone, or some small group of people, attain freedom from their particular disease. On the other hand, there appears to be no scientifically controlled double-blind studies that clearly point to a particular diet to cure cancer or a specific cancer, for example. How much of these dietary successes is due to the placebo effect? Probably a significant amount, but only a proper study will say how much. Otherwise, the evidence is anecdotal and word-of-mouth.

Are there particular diets or dietary guidelines that are effective? In the next chapter, H. Ira Fritz, Ph.D., who is a specialist in nutrition, gives his considered opinion on diets for those with life-challenging diseases. Are his views the last word? No. But, they are a reasoned set of recommendations based on his careful study of the literature. Andrew Weil, M.D. has written (1972, 1995, 1996) sensibly about nutrition. A common-sense approach towards nutrition means eating a balanced diet with plenty of fresh fruits and vegetables, and a minimum of processed, fried or fatty foods. The odds are on your side if you do not smoke, over-eat, over-drink, or vegetate as a couch potato.

Most of the special diets start with a 'body cleansing' routine that involves lots of water and/or fresh fruit juices, fasting, and something like a brown rice diet for a week or two. Coffee enemas are sometimes recommended as a way of 'detoxifying' the body. You should consult your physician before attempting a cleansing/detoxifying regimen.

Figure 5.12: Reading product claims in a health food store.

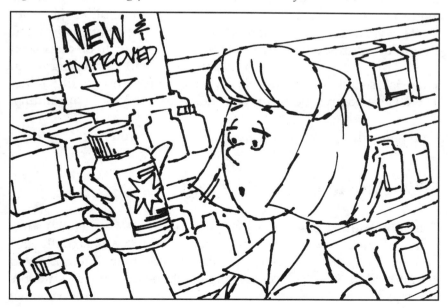

101

Under the heading of 'nutrition' can be added a seemingly endless array of food supplements. These include: antioxidants, vitamins, Essiac tea, the Hoxie herbal solution, amino acids, B complexes, coenzyme Q10, and vitamin C, which all have their adherents. *If* the side-effects are minimal, you may wish to cautiously explore these supplements. The discipline required to follow a particular diet or set of supplements may be too restrictive or uncomfortable for you and your lifestyle. Before you commit to a dietary/supplement regimen, check and double-check. Also, consult your physician.

There are special nutritional considerations for people who are in the last stage of their life. At this stage, eating is a quality-of-life issue that *may or may not need* to be balanced with 'good nutrients.' At this stage, you may have weakness, be too tired to eat, have anorexia from the disease or drug regimens, have nausea and vomiting from the disease or drugs, have tissue breakdown in your mouth that makes eating uncomfortable and/or have depression that leads to loss of appetite, and you may have difficulty in swallowing due to neurological involvement, etc. These are hard things to cope with both for you, your caregivers, and helping professionals. Since families tend to see eating as a sign of hope, they may insist on an aggressive nutritional program, as this often implies a curative treatment program for them. Of course, the amounts and kinds of food become important—comfort foods tend to be of the breakfast variety and may not be older 'favorite' foods. Hydration, natural and artificial, is an important aspect and should be addressed. Nutrition at this stage needs to be discussed openly by you, your family, and your professional helping team. There is a search for a balance between quantity and quality of life, as well as a balance between your needs and those of your family.

If you are what you eat, be careful about what you eat.

5.17 *Physical Exercise*

The book entitled *Biomarkers* by Evans and Rosenberg (1992) summarizes much exercise physiology research that was actually carried out with and for older people, rather than attempting to extrapolate the results of experiments made with college students as subjects. Their message is simple—it is never too late to change your diet and/or the amount and kind of exercise. Evans and Rosenberg (1992, p. 42) indicate that there are 10 biomarkers of vitality that *you can alter*. They are:

1. Your muscle mass
2. Your strength
3. Your basal metabolic rate (BMR)
4. Your body fat percentage
5. Your aerobic capacity
6. Your body's blood sugar tolerance
7. Your cholesterol/HDL (high-density lipid) ratio
8. Your blood pressure
9. Your bone density
10. Your body's ability to regulate its internal temperature

Each of these 10 items is discussed extensively. Their book gives a detailed program for these 10 biomarkers that is specifically designed for the older population, but is also relevant to younger populations and those with diseases. Nutrition was covered briefly in the last section and in more detail in the next chapter. Exercise falls into three categories: aerobic, anaerobic, and weight-bearing. First, we will discuss some general aspects of exercise.

Aerobic exercises are done at a rate that allows sufficient oxygen to get to tissues. They are fast-paced activities that make you huff and puff. They place demands on your cardiovascular apparatus. *Anaerobic* exercises are so strenuous that the tissues end up with an oxygen deficiency. *Anaerobic* activities are those like sprinting, where the body can do 'without oxygen' for a short period of time. You should exercise only in the aerobic range. Bailey (1991) points out that exercises like jogging need to be done at such a rate that you have sufficient wind to talk with a fellow jogger. Exercises that involve the large muscles in the legs are more effective than upper body exercises that involve smaller muscles. Thus, jogging, biking, fast walking, stepping machines, and cross-country skiing (or ski machines) are more useful than swimming, which is mainly an upper body exercise. Three to four sessions per week of aerobic exercise that last at least 30 minutes appear to be the minimum to maintain fitness. For older people, probably the best exercise (less strain on joints) is vigorous walking. Start with what you can do now, even if it is only 100 feet, and extend your range and speed a little bit each day.

Consistency is important. Stretching before *and* after exercising reduces strain. Start your exercise session with a five- to 10-minute low-intensity aerobic warm-up, followed by five minutes of stretching. End your activity with five to 10 minutes of an aerobic cool-down, slowing down gradually, and follow by stretching.

Working out in a weight room has two effects: building muscle mass and increasing bone density. The authors of *Biomarkers* point out that muscle improvement is highly specific. An exercise to strengthen your right biceps will strengthen only your right biceps. So, a weight room regimen involves a variety of machines or free weights so that all principal muscle groups are exercised. You work with a particular muscle group and weight doing up to 12 repetitions (reps) before fatiguing. If you can do only a few reps with a particular weight, then go to a lower weight. When it is easy to do 12 or more reps, go to the next highest weight. Do not exceed 80% of your maximal capacity to lift. Avoid locking elbow or knee joints when lifting. Recent research suggests that one set of 12 reps done two to three times each week is sufficient to maintain and even extend fitness. Muscles grow in a particular pattern in response to stressing them. They increase in mass over a 24- to 36-hour period. So, exercise a particular muscle group no more frequently than *every other day*. If you wish to use the weight room daily, then alternate muscle groups each day.

The way the body increases bone mass works differently than for muscle mass. Apparently, according to the *Biomarkers* researchers (see pp. 77–81), weight-bearing exercises for *any* bone or bone group in the body signals the body to uniformly increase bone mass in *all* of the bones in the body. So, *any* kind of weight-bearing exercise is important for older people to strengthen their bones *throughout* their bodies, that is, there is a whole-body effect. These exercises can begin, even for bed-ridden people, by doing something simple like raising a paperback book a dozen times, two to three times each day. They can then progress to heavier paperbacks and other objects.

This section on exercise may appear to be irrelevant for someone who has a life-challenging disease. Since you can derive benefit from both aerobic and weight-bearing exercise at almost any stage of a disease, it is worth knowing about exercise and being involved in some exercise activity, even if bed-ridden. There is an almost immediate positive feedback from exercise, which encourages you

Figure 5.13a&b: Aerobic exercise and weight training.

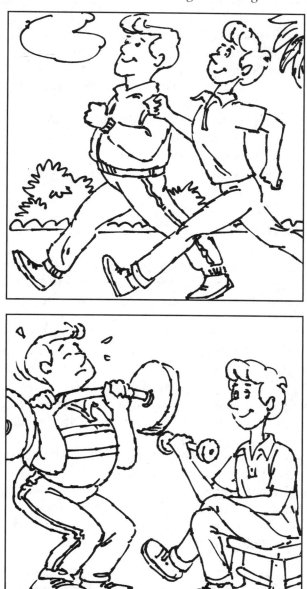

to do more. In addition to this physical sense, there is the more important feeling of control, doing something that makes you feel good and strengthens you. So, consider doing some exercise that you can do on a regular basis.

5.18 Acupuncture

Many people get relief from acupuncture treatments. The paper by Melzack, Stillwell, and Fox (1977) provides a potential scientific basis for the use of acupuncture. Acupuncture has been used for pain control, for nausea and vomiting related to chemotherapy, and to alleviate the side-effects due to radiation treatment. When seeking an acupuncturist, consult with knowledgeable people, and work with someone who has been in the field for a significant length of time, like 10 years or more. This is a treatment where the years of experience of the practitioner are important. There are licensed acupuncturists.

5.19 Hypnosis

Hypnosis has much to offer in a variety of ways. For example, hypnosis is well-established as a method of pain control. There are no side-effects, and the patient can generally be quite sentient. Hypnosis can be used to control the nausea that often accompanies chemotherapy treatments. It can also help to minimize the side-effects of radiotherapy treatments. Hypnosis generally has a calming and relaxing effect. Guided imagery work can be considered a kind of hypnosis since hypnotic language skills are needed for effective work. Hypnosis has also been used to prepare people for surgery and other invasive treatments. (See Battino, 2000.)

Many hospitals now have a hypnotherapist on staff, or on their list of consultants. At the worst, hypnosis will be of little help; at the best, of significant help; but, there are also no side-effects. The American Society of Clinical Hypnosis can provide referrals (847-297-3317). The Milton H. Erickson Foundation also provides referrals (602-956-6196).

5.20 Talking to a Comatose Patient

Just as there is evidence that people under the surgical plane of anesthesia can hear and understand what is said to them (for example, see Pearson, 1961; Rossi and Cheek, 1988, pp. 113–130; and Bank, 1985), there are also strong indications that people in comas can hear and respond on some level to what is said to them. At the minimum, it helps the person doing the talking—they can express their concern and love and feel that they are communicating with a loved one. Physical contact, like holding a hand, appears to help this communication. It is similarly important to talk to people who have had strokes or amyotrophic lateral sclerosis and who are limited in the ways they can respond. You can read poetry, favorite passages, or entire books. You can ask for responses like eye blinks or hand squeezes. Although it is sometimes hard to do this kind of communicating, for some people it is very satisfying.

5.21 Grieving

Your survivors will grieve for you—there is also grieving to be done by you before that time. To grieve is to acknowledge a loss—that loss can be of a person, a pet, a favorite object, and missed opportunities. Saying goodbye to life and all it has meant to you can be helped by consciously grieving over your losses. This is not something that needs to be done to excess with great wailings and gnashings of teeth. It is generally done with some sadness, some nostalgia, and many good memories. If this kind of grieving and letting go makes sense to you, then do it privately or with someone you trust. As discussed earlier in the section on ceremonies, you may wish to devise a ceremony for grieving. We are all somewhat saddened by losses, even anticipated losses, and buoyed up by happy memories. Taking time to grieve in anticipation of loss is difficult but beneficial, whether it is for your own life, for things left undone, for people or things left behind, or for all of these for a loved one. It is a letting go with appreciation and nostalgia, a natural clearing of the way. Brooks (1985) has written a remarkable book on grieving the loss of her husband—the book is in the form of a monthly journal (see Section 4.3 for a structured writing workbook for grieving).

5.22 Meditation and Relaxation

How do you relax given the continuing stress and interruptions to your life that a serious disease brings about? If you are already adept at meditation or doing self-relaxation, then you need to *schedule* one or two fixed times each day for this purpose. The word 'schedule' is emphasized since for healing—and curing—relaxation may be as important as treatments. It is said, for example, that the *panic reaction* that accompanies a heart attack kills more people than the physical damage to the heart. In this regard, it is enlightening to read how Norman Cousins (1984) handled his heart attack. To lower his tension level, and the tension level of those around him, he told jokes to by-standers and the paramedics who took him to the hospital!

There are many relaxation/meditation tapes available. There are courses in how to meditate and relax. Your therapist or a friend could make a relaxation tape for you. You can make such a tape for yourself by taping one of the many available scripts, or favorite passages from the Bible, Koran, Torah, Vedas, books of poetry, etc.

Most people find a long soak in a hot bath, or a long shower, to be very relaxing. You know the things that you do that are most relaxing for you. This may be music or a good book or watching television or going out with friends or the theater or the movies. Note that the effectiveness of your immune system is enhanced when you are in a relaxed state.

Figure 5.14: Relaxing and meditating.

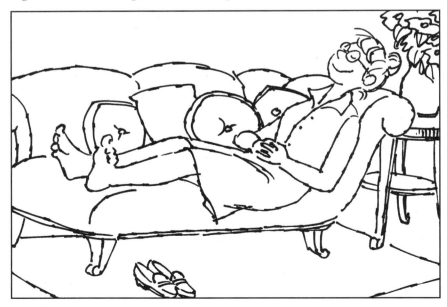

5.23 *Ideomotor Signaling*

One way to cope with the changes going on in your body and all the new sensations is to use ideomotor signaling to query your body's inner sense of what is going on. If you are good at this technique, it can be of great use to you in assessing what goes on in your body. It does take practice, and an experienced hypnotherapist can get you started and teach you what you need to know. Alternatively, you may just go to a hypnotist and have him/her guide you through this kind of body scan.

It has been said, 'The body never lies.' and 'Who knows your body better than you?' Ideomotor finger signaling is one way to put these two observations together. Some information on this follows.

Automatic or non-volitional movements are called *ideomotor* or *ideodynamic*. Ideomotor signals are used as a way to query your own mind/body about what is going on in it. They have also been used for some time (Rossi and Cheek, 1988; Cheek, 1994) to elicit responses from the inner or unconscious mind. The parlor games of the Ouija board and automatic writing involve ideomotor movements, i.e., micromuscular movements that are apparently not under conscious control. The Chevreul pendulum, a light weight hanging from a thread or fine chain, has been used to indicate responses to questions. These questions are designed to obtain three responses: "yes," "no," and "I'm not ready to answer now." (The third response used to be "maybe," until it was recognized just how lazy the inner mind is, i.e., this was the most frequent answer!)

Figure 5.15: Finger signals. "Yes," "No," and "I'm not ready to answer now."

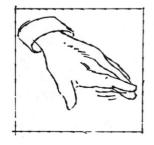 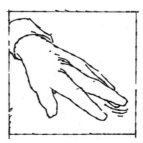 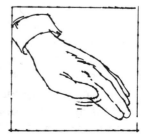

Once you have learned to get into a relaxed or meditative state, and can do this for 15 to 20 minutes, then you can practice using ideo-motor finger signals to ask your own body questions. In the relaxed state, ask your inner mind to designate a "yes" finger, that is, one that will move when you internally ask a question whose obvious answer is "yes." Then, do the same to establish a "no" finger, and an "I do not wish to answer now" finger. These automatic finger movements are typically small and jerky. If you have cancer, either active or in remission, or some other serious ailment, you probably get overly concerned about new pains and aches and discomforts. Is it the cancer recurring or spreading, or is that pain a muscle strain or gas or something else that is temporary and not serious? In the relaxed state, you can query your body about the significance of a particular pain or discomfort. "Should I see the doctor about this?" "Is this serious?" "Will it pass normally?" When you are adept at this kind of finger signaling, it makes it easier to live with changing conditions. But, it does take practice to become proficient. As indicated above, a hypnotist can teach you how to use this interesting method for yourself. Always check with your physician if you are in doubt about what your fingers tell you.

5.24 *Simplicity*

The *simplicity* movement has been growing in the U.S. The goal is to simplify your life. In a consumer society driven by advertising, we are continually urged to buy more and more things. A personal computer that was state-of-the-art three years ago is considered to be obsolete technology today—too slow and too little memory. How often do you replace your car, your washing machine, your vacuum cleaner, your stereo equipment, etc.? Do you really need another pair of shoes? Can you share a lawn mower with your neighbor? With several neighbors? How much 'stuff' do you really need?

When you are diagnosed with a life-challenging disease or have some catastrophic event in your life, you suddenly get a different perspective on what things are really important. These are your health and your relationships. 'Objects' no longer have the same value. That promotion you were 'killing yourself for' is literally not worth dying—or living—for. Don't wait for cancer for permission to find meaning in your life. Don't wait to begin simplifying your life.

Figure 5.16a&b: Keep it simple!

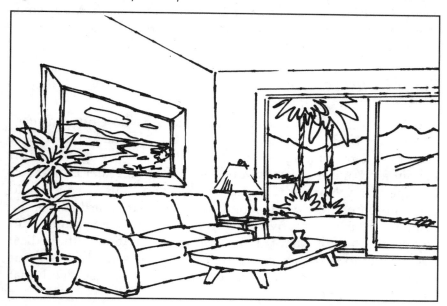

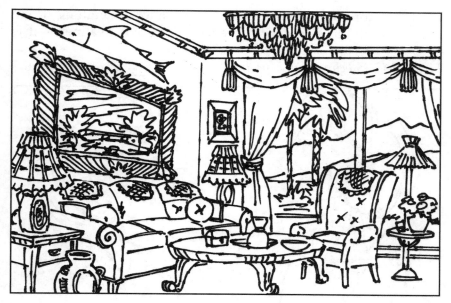

There are several good books (Elgin, 1981; St. James, 1994; Andrews, 1997; Luhrs, 1997) on simplicity. The titles of these four books, respectively, are illuminating: *Voluntary simplicity. Toward a way of life that is outwardly simple, inwardly rich; Simplify your life. 100 ways*

to slow down and enjoy the things that really matter; *The circle of simplicity. Return to the good life*; and *The simple living guide*. Many communities have simplicity circles and study groups.

5.25 *Laughter*

The *Reader's Digest* has a long-standing feature whose title is, *Laughter—the Best Medicine*. When was the last time you had a *belly* laugh, one of those fits of laughter that brings tears to your eyes, a stitch in your side, and has you fighting for breath? Laughter is an excellent medicine. Norman Cousins (1979) literally used laughter to cure himself of ankylosing spondylitis, rheumatoid arthritis of the spine where the connective tissue progressively disintegrates with no known cause or cure. He did this in collaboration with medical advice. We do know from David Spiegel et al.'s work (1989) that mental attitudes can have profound physical effects, and that laughter is healing.

In many support group meetings, there is a lot of laughing. There is occasional 'black' humor related to disease or treatment—it is

Figure 5.17: A belly laugh is healing.

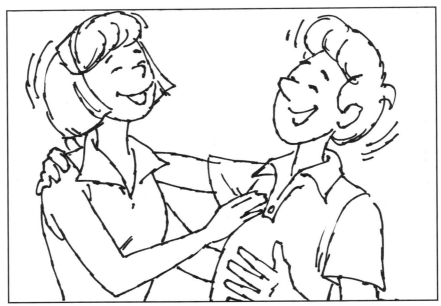

really only occasional. People simply enjoy laughing together. People bring in jokes and cartoons to share. The world outside of the support group is too serious. Aside from Patch Adams (1998), how many doctors are willing to clown it up? Families frequently feel it is inappropriate to laugh or do fun things—he's got cancer, you know. If what you are doing isn't FUN, what is it? If you can't laugh, can you be alive? Laugh and the world laughs with you. Crying alone is sad. The studies probably haven't been done yet, but I am willing to bet that the immune system is enhanced by laughter. Since you can't physiologically be panicked and relaxed at the same time, which one will you choose?

I heard a joke the other day ...

5.26 Dying Well

Dying well takes some planning, some thinking, much cooperation, and some luck. Have you thought about your last days? What you would like them to be like? How would you realize that dream? Yes, we may have no control over that event or its timing, but we can

Figure 5.18: Dying well—at home with your family.

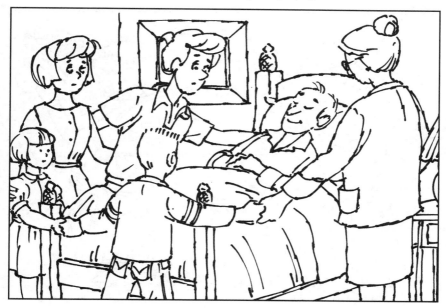

dream and hope and plan. This is a natural event, and can be joyous, a celebration of life, of accomplishments, of love. It is good to do some planning about your last hours or days well in advance. If you have specific desires or wishes, let your family know, and even write them out. Do you prefer to die at home? In your own bed? With which of your loved ones in attendance? With music and of what kind? With a priest/rabbi/minister in attendance? In a room full of flowers and special photographs or paintings? Holding hands together? Singing a special hymn? Reciting a special prayer? Hugging, kissing, or touching everyone? Or alone with your own thoughts? Let your preferences be known. These are your choices, and you can die well, and in your own way.

5.27 *Living Well*

It has been said that the 'best revenge' on people who have given you negative or 'witch' messages, or who wish you ill, or whose expectations for you are low and full of gloom and doom, is to *live well*, to live your life as if it were the only one you have, to make

Figure 5.19: Living well.

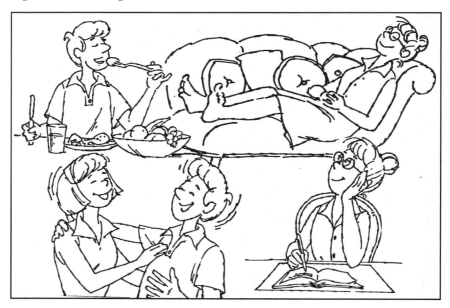

each moment count, to succeed in whatever has meaning for you. In a sense we are all dying from the moment of our birth—some of us take longer than others. We are all 'terminal' since we will all die—the date and the time is uncertain even for last-stage patients. So, why not *live* until that inevitable moment? To be alive means that you are making choices, taking risks (not crazy ones!), exploring, being in the moment, really tasting and touching and smelling and seeing and hearing—doing all of this *now* rather than postponing to the future or resurrecting from the past. Do not wait for a catastrophic diagnosis to activate your life and senses. Get in all of the living you can at this moment. Live well.

5.28 Doka's Phases of a Life-Challenging Disease

Doka (1993) suggests that there are four to five phases of a life-challenging disease: prediagnostic, acute, chronic, (recovery), and terminal. He then suggests that there are a number of tasks that are characteristic of each phase. These tasks and some comments about each phase follow, and are based on Doka's book, pp. 6–11. It may be helpful to you to know about these phases and their characteristics. Or, you may just wish to skip this section.

Figure 5.20: The phases of a life-challenging disease. (Patterned after Doka, 1993, p. 6.)

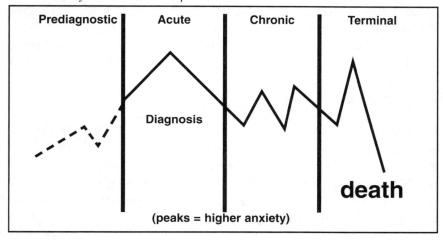

115

a. *Prediagnostic Phase*. This often precedes diagnosis, and is a time when a person recognizes symptoms or risk factors that might make him prone to disease. The tasks for coping with such a potential threat include:

- Recognizing possible danger or risks.
- Coping with anxiety and uncertainty.
- Developing and following through on a health-seeking strategy.

b. *Acute Phase*. This centers around the crisis of diagnosis. Once the diagnosis has been made of a life-challenging disease, there are a number of decisions—medical, psychological, interpersonal, financial—that need to be made to cope with this crisis. Tasks include:

- Understanding the disease.
- Examining and maximizing health and lifestyle.
- Maximizing one's coping strengths and limiting weakness.
- Examining internal and external resources and liabilities.
- Developing strategies to deal with the issues created by the disease (coping with professionals, interpersonal relationships, treatment options, financial matters, etc.).
- Exploring the effect of the disease on one's sense of self and relationships with others; also exploring spiritual values.
- Venting feelings and fears.
- Integrating the reality of the diagnosis with one's past life and future plans.

c. *Chronic Phase*. During this time, the individual is actively struggling with the disease, its treatment, and all related concerns. Within the constraints of the disease, many people successfully lead normal or close-to-normal lives. However, this time is punctuated by disease-related crises. Tasks in this phase would include:

- Managing symptoms and side-effects.
- Carrying out health regimens.
- Preventing and managing health crises.
- Managing stress and examining coping.
- Maximizing social support and minimizing isolation.
- Normalizing life within the constraints of the disease.
- Dealing with financial concerns, including medical insurance.
- Preserving self-concept.

- Redefining relationships with others throughout the course of the disease.
- Venting feelings and fears.
- Finding meaning in suffering, chronicity, uncertainty, and decline.

d. *Recovery Phase*. This may not appear, or it may be a permanent recovery—really long-term remission, or there may be a series of recoveries of varying duration. Some of the tasks in a recovery phase are:

- Dealing with psychological, social, physical, spiritual, and financial after-effects of the disease.
- Coping with fears and anxieties about recurrence.
- Examining life and lifestyle issues and reconstructing one's life.
- Redefining relationships with caregivers.

e. *Terminal Phase*. This is the phase where the disease has progressed to the point where death is inevitable. Death is now likely rather than possible or probable. Death then becomes the individual's and the family's central crisis. Tasks at this time include:

- Dealing with symptoms, discomfort, pain, and incapacitation.
- Managing health and institutional procedures.
- Managing stress and examining coping.
- Dealing effectively with caregivers.
- Preparing for death and saying good-byes.
- Preserving self-concept.
- Preserving appropriate relationships with family and friends.
- Dealing with unfinished business as appropriate and within capabilities.
- Venting feelings and fears.
- Finding meaning in life and death; exploring spiritual life.

With respect to these phases and their associated tasks, Doka (p. 11, 1993) has the following to add: "Life-threatening illness is inevitably family illness, for the life of everyone within the family is changed when one member of a family experiences disease." A wise man, and a helpful book.

5.29 *Hammerschlag's Recommendations*

Carl Hammerschlag's recommendations for staying healthy and curing disease are a good way to end this chapter. (You may read the complete annotated list at his website, which also contains other useful information, including links to health sites, e.g., www.healingdoc.com.)

- Be positive and celebrate life.
- Appreciate your own uniqueness and self worth.
- Recognize that adversity is part of life and deal with it in a positive way.
- Take action.
- Make choices.
- Train your unconscious mind.
- Take care of your unfinished business.
- Heal your spirit.
- Deal with fear.
- Look at your life differently.
- Live in the present.
- Trust your intuition.
- Listen to your heart.
- Be consistent in thought, word, and deed.
- Let go of anger.
- Look to serve others.
- Become a visionary.
- Love others and seek love in return.
- Believe and have faith.
- Pray.

I would add to this list: be sure to have fun and laugh a lot.

5.30 *Summary*

This chapter gives information on the many ways you can cope with the system and take care of yourself. You always have the choice about what you think and feel about a situation. There is much more that is under your control than you think. The extremes are: being a passive person that things are *done to*; or an active agent that things are *done by and with*. The more control you have over your life and treatment, the better the odds for a good outcome. Enjoy!

Chapter Six
Nutrition and Life-Challenging Diseases

H. Ira Fritz, Ph.D.

6.1 Introduction: Lifestyle and an Integrated Approach

Eating is a basic part of life. The science of nutrition deals with the effect of food on health and well-being. However, there is much variation by both the lay public and health professionals on what should be eaten in what quantities. In this chapter there are some recommendations on diets for the prevention of disease, and for controlling or curing a disease. Diet cannot be considered solely by itself, but needs to be part of a total lifestyle program. An *integrated* approach to health includes, in addition to proper nutrition: a regular exercise program of both the aerobic and resistance type, attention to group support and social networks, and attention to relaxation. A balanced diet should involve eating within your cultural traditions, and include a wide variety of primarily wholefoods. Nutrition cannot be considered just by itself, nor by focusing on a single disease.

6.2 Prevention

In this section three nutritional approaches are discussed: (1) the U.S. Department of Agriculture's *Food Pyramid*; (2) the Ornish diet and its related activities; and (3) the Traditional Healthy Mediterranean Diet Pyramid.

On the chemoprevention of cancer, it appears safe to recommend a varied diet that is consistent with the U.S. Department of

Agriculture's *Food Pyramid*. They recommend three to five servings of vegetables and two to four servings of fruits each day. There is good evidence that the consistent consumption of fruits and vegetables is protective against cancer. Fiber consumption reduces the risk of both cardiovascular disease and gastrointestinal cancers. The results vary with the type of fiber. Soluble fiber found in oat bran, fruit pectins, and legumes seems to be involved in cardiovascular health. Insoluble fiber found in wheat bran, wholegrain breads and cereals, and vegetables seems to be preventative for colon cancer. There are some specific vitamins and minerals that have been studied. Generally, they are antioxidants. In one study (Clark, et al., 1996), it was found that 200 mcg (micrograms) per day of orally supplemented selenium had a preventative effect on certain types of cancer. Folic acid (also called folate) at 400 mcg per day was found to reduce the risk of pancreatic cancer in men and breast cancer in women. Linus Pauling, among others, suggested the widespread use of vitamin C. The evidence seems inconclusive. Although beta-carotene (a precursor of vitamin A) has been suggested as being useful because it is present in many fruits and vegetables, the results of a large study in Finland showed an increased risk of cancer with beta-carotene consumption. Lycopene and lutein are related to beta-carotene and have been suggested as being beneficial. Materials called bioflavonoids and polyphenols can also serve as antioxidants and seem to have preventative effects. Some examples of foods that contain these compounds are green tea and grapes (especially the seeds).

For the prevention of cardiovascular disease, the situation is more complicated. Low-fat diets help, as does an intake of antioxidants. Exercise is important. The daily intake of a small amount of alcohol (4–6 ounces of wine, 12 ounces of beer, or 1.5 ounces of distilled spirit) appears to help, as does the daily taking of one-quarter of a standard 325-mg aspirin pill.

The Ornish (1991) intervention program for the reversal of heart disease involves several parts. There is a low-fat vegetarian diet, an exercise program (walking is recommended), programmed relaxation, and group interaction and support. Although Ornish believes that diet is the key to reversing atherosclerotic 'clogging,' he acknowledges (and his published work supports) that it is the *combination* of all of the parts of his program that makes it effective.

Diet is just one part, and it is not clear what is its contribution to the whole. Eating and food preparation have social as well as nutritional significance.

Figure 6.1: The Traditional Healthy Mediterranean Diet Pyramid (reprinted with permission of the Oldways Preservation and Exchange Trust).

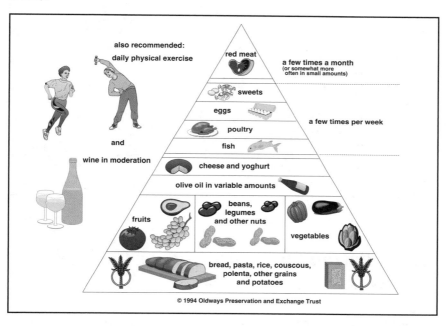

The Traditional Healthy Mediterranean Diet Pyramid (Gifford, 1998) is shown above. The base of this pyramid is whole grains and other starches. Fruits, vegetables and legumes are the next level, and are followed by olive oil, cheese and yogurt (low-fat varieties are recommended). Animal protein is represented by fish and poultry, with limited amounts of eggs and desserts, and very limited amounts of red meat. There is evidence that this easy-to-follow nutritional regimen may decrease the risk of cardiovascular disease. Gifford (1998) suggests that the preparation and consumption of food are important social events. This supports Ornish's idea that group interaction is an important part of cardiovascular health.

Figure 6.2: Eating well and healthily.

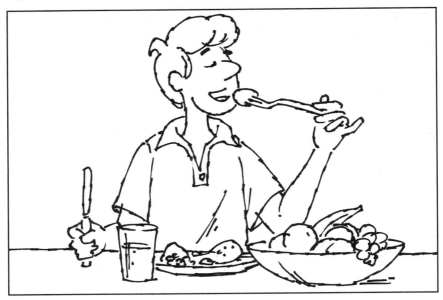

6.3 *Nutrition for Controlling or Curing a Disease*

There are two major nutritional issues when one is ill. The first is getting enough nutrients to help the body resist/fight the disease, and the second is not eating foods that make the disease worse. In many illnesses, the desire for food is quickly lost. Every effort should be made to increase food consumption. Frequent, small meals of favorite foods is one approach. Another thing to try is to use some type of appetite stimulant. There is a volatile oil in onions that seems to be effective. Sautéing onions just before a meal usually increases food intake. There is another notion that I think is important. I generally ask my classes, "*Why* do you eat?" The answers fall into three categories: feelings (let's celebrate with a hot fudge sundae, let's drown our sorrows in a hot fudge sundae), social reasons (this is the time all my friends eat, I went over to my neighbors for a cup of coffee and ...) and physiology (i.e., hunger). It is important to realize that hunger is only one of the reasons that we eat. The social setting and the interaction of friends and family around food is extremely important and needs to be taken into consideration when dealing with the appetite of someone who is ill.

For cardiovascular disease, the work of Ornish (1991) has shown dramatically that atherosclerotic lesions (plaques) can be reversed, and that the risk of occlusive cardiovascular disease can be decreased. But, Ornish believes you have to *adhere rigorously* to the suggested diet *and* include the other lifestyle changes.

With respect to cancer, the results of changing eating patterns is less promising, although there are many proponents of specific dietary regimens. There is no convincing evidence in the literature supporting diet as an adjunct in cancer treatment. Certainly, a balanced eating plan, such as one based on the Mediterranean Food Pyramid, improves general well-being.

There are a number of supplements that can be useful. Some source of omega-3 fatty acids (fish oils or flaxseed oil) should be in your diet. Antioxidants such as vitamin E (300-600 IU per day, and preferably the natural form), vitamin C (up to 1.5–2.0 g per day appears to be safe), selenium (a total of 50–100 mcg per day), and calcium (about 1000 mg/day, and 1500 mg/day for postmenopausal women susceptible to osteoporosis). If you take calcium as a supplement, you also need to take magnesium, with a calcium-to-magnesium ratio of about 2.25–3 to 1. Minerals are generally best taken with food.

6.4 Summary

A healthy diet such as the Mediterranean one promotes general well-being and health. There is a diet that can considerably help with cardiovascular disease. There is no comparable diet for any of the cancers. Wise dietary choices can help prevent serious disease. Eat wisely and well and, as far as possible, in a way that also gives you enjoyment.

For those interested in more detailed information on nutrition and serious diseases, four comprehensive sources are cited here. These are all well-researched volumes with specialty chapters written by experts in the field. You may wish to inform your oncologist and physician about these materials and resources. The first is a 1990 publication (Bloch, 1990) on nutrition management of the cancer patient. In addition to general information, there is specific information on nutritional needs for the various cancers. The volume edited by Matarese and Gottschlich (1998) is entitled *Contemporary Nutrition Support Practice. A Clinical Guide.* There are many chapters by experts on nutrition related to specific diseases like: neurological impairment; cardiac, pulmonary, hepatic, and renal failure; gastrointestinal and pancreatic disease; and cancer. The Cancer Treatment Research Foundation has sponsored a special book on *Nutritional Oncology* (Heber, Blackburn, Go, 1999). This book contains specialty chapters on nutrition for many forms of cancer. Section II is on nutrition and the etiology (origins) of cancer; and Section III is on diet, nutrition, and cancer prevention. Section V discusses clinical trials in nutritional oncology. A recent volume (Bloch, 2000) is for the physician and contains "a comprehensive collection of patient education handouts and practitioner resources that: helps you customize individual patient education programs, helps answer questions on basic nutrition and the side effects of cancer treatment; supplies special diets for immediate use; and provides materials in English and Spanish and at two literacy levels." Your oncologist should know about this book.

Chapter Seven
Beyond Coping

The word 'coping' implies putting up with things in your life that you cannot change. You are stuck, life has dealt you a lousy hand, and how do you live with it? Yet, the thesis of this book is that there are many many ways to respond to adversity. You always have the choice of your attitude, how you react. Do you just give up and accept your fate, or do you rally and fight, doing everything within your power to live your life as fully as you can at this moment? Is your life half empty or half full? You always have choices. You might even say that being alive has to do with choosing. Norman Cousins chose to joke rather than panic when he had his heart attack. He chose to postpone a stress test because the ambiance was negative for him. He chose to laugh *and* work with his doctors when he was diagnosed with an incurable disease. You are what you choose.

The coping skills discussed here have to do with your making choices, and taking charge of your own life and treatment. To be sure, it is wise to consult experienced and skilled professionals in making these decisions. Yet, it is your life, your quality of life, that is at stake when you take charge. And, there is much more that is under your control than you might first imagine. Chapters Four and Five list many of these items. Feeling out of control leads to a sense of helplessness, then hopelessness and despair, even depression. Taking charge of even the smallest aspects of your life is an act of hope, an assertion of your individuality, a recognition of yourself as a valued person. So, take charge now—it is an important part, perhaps the essential part, of your healing journey.

Finally, I want to thank you for sharing part of your life with me. Everyone is unique and individual and exceptional. Peace *and* Love *and* Healing.

Appendix A

Questions for People in their Dying Time

Lawrence LeShan has compiled a list of 33 significant questions for people in their dying time to consider (1989, pp. 161–165). These are good questions to ponder at any time of your life. You may find these questions to be useful in organizing your thinking and considering your life. You may wish to share your responses with a compassionate friend or relative, or write your responses in your journal.

1. As you look at your whole life from the viewpoint of where you are now, what was it all about? Was it a good life? Was it a lonely life? Was it a frustrating life?
2. If your whole life had been designed in advance so that you would learn something from it, what would be the lesson you were supposed to have learned? Did you really learn it? What else would you have needed in order to have learned it?
3. What was the best thing that ever happened to you? What was the worst? (These are separate questions and, as a general rule, seem to be the most helpful when asked in this order.)
4. What was the best thing you ever did? What was the worst?
5. What was the best period of your life? What was the worst?
6. How would you finish these statements: "Out of my childhood I love to remember ..." "Out of my childhood I hate to remember ..."?
7. Do you believe it is true that "It is better to have loved and lost than never to have loved at all"? What led you to this conclusion?
8. If you were asked by a child you love to tell him or her the one most important thing that you have learned in life, what would you reply?
9. There is an old Greek legend about the three Fates who govern all lives: Clotho, who weaves the thread of a person's life; Lachesis, who colors it; and Atropos, who cuts it and the person dies. How did Lachesis color *your* life? Did Atropos cut it off too soon? Too soon for what? Can you still do what you have left unfinished so far?

10. In each symphony (ballad, folksong, popular song) there is a central theme. It has many variations, these appear in the different sections (verses), but underlying them all is the theme. What has been the theme of your life?
11. If you could change *one decision* of your life, what would it be? Why did you make it the way you did? What does this tell you about how you saw yourself and the world at that time? Can you forgive yourself for making that decision the way you did? For feeling the way you did? If not, why?
12. For the things you did, what do you now need to do in order to be able to forgive yourself?
13. For the things that others did to you, what do you need to do in order to forgive them? For the things that happened to you, what do you need in order to forgive yourself?
14. If you were to overhear your friends talking about you at your funeral, what would you most like to hear them say about you? Like least to hear?
15. As you look back on your life, what were the moments when you were most yourself? What helped you to do this? What were the moments you were least yourself? Why do you think this was so?
16. What was the best time of your life? Tell me about it? What was the worst time of your life? Tell me about it.
17. How were you the same all your life, as a child, a youth, an adult, now? How were you different at those different times of your life?
18. What do you need to finish your life, to complete it? Can you do it from this hospital room?
19. During this time, what is the longest time of the day for you? What do you mostly feel and think during this time?
20. In an ancient manuscript *The Book of Splendor* is the statement: "God's purpose is not to add years to your life, but to add life to your years." What do you think of this?
21. What is the thing in yourself that you have been most afraid to experience consciously? To think and feel about? Does it now seem as necessary to hide it from yourself as it did in the past?
22. What is it about you that you have most hidden from others? Does it seem as necessary to keep it hidden as it did in the past?
23. All our lives we try to change people to what we think they should be. At this time of life we can often see that love is accepting people as they are and letting them be while hoping

and wishing for more for them. Can you do this with those you love? What in you keeps you from this?

24. The time of dying is the last learning time we have on Earth. What lesson is there for you to learn in your dying? What in you keeps you from being able to learn it?

25. What is the major role you have played in recent years? What masks have you worn most often in the presence of others? Are they roles you wish to play during these last times?

26. All our lives we try to *accomplish* something, to *do* something. What is it that you were trying to do in recent years? Is it still so important to you? How can you finish the attempt so that it ends with the most harmony and honesty?

27. Have you been mostly walking one road in recent years? Is there another road that you now need to walk in order to make your life journey more complete?

28. Is there someone you protected in recent years at a high cost in energy and time? Are you still trying to protect him or her? (Or be something for him or her?) Is it the best thing for this person for you to continue protecting him or her? For you?

29. What do you need to *finish* your life? Can you do it from this bed? How or why not? It is in *you* that we need to finish things and it is inside you that you can.

30. What is it that has happened to you that you have never been able to forgive God (or the Fates) for?

31. For what do you most need the forgiveness of God?

32. There is the story of one of the great Hasidic Rabbis named Zusya. His congregation asked him to do something, a particular political action. He refused. They said, "If Moses were our Rabbi, he would do it." Zusya answered, "When I die and rise and stand before the throne, God will not ask me why I was not Moses. He will ask me why I was not Zusya." Does this story in any way relate to you and your life? How?

33. What has been the best season of the year for you? Why?

Appendix B

Some Relevant Websites and Phone Numbers

Websites

The following are a few of the enormous number of websites that I have found to be useful. Searching the Web under the key words of 'imagery,' 'guided imagery,' and 'cancer,' for example, will send you off on an exploration of many sources of information, as well as much vending of particular products and services. OncoLink is a very good place to start your search for information on cancer. Also listed are websites for several other serious diseases. There are phone numbers for many of these organizations at the end of this appendix. The following list is in alphabetical order.

Academy for Guided Imagery, Inc.
www.healthy.com/agi

Aging With Dignity—Has prepared the "Five Wishes" document.
www.agingwithdignity.org

Alternative Therapies in Health and Medicine—This is the premier journal in the field.
www.alternative-therapies.com/select/currentmain.html

American Cancer Society—Information in many categories including living with cancer and treatments.
www.cancer.org

American Heart Association—Their basic website on diseases of the heart.
www.americanheart.org

American Society of Clinical Oncology—People Living With Cancer Section—Special information by oncologists for those with cancer.
www.asco.org

Amyotrophic Lateral Sclerosis (ALS) or Motor Neurone Disease (MND), also known in the U.S.A. as Lou Gehrig's Disease—This site is the "ALS Survival Guide."
www.lougehrigsdisease.net

Arbor Nutrition Guide—An excellent source about nutrition in general, which contains many categories and has links to other sources. Of special interest may be the section on vegetarian and alternative nutrition, also with many links.
www.arbor.nutrition.com

Bloch Cancer Foundation—The Website of the Bloch Cancer Foundation lists many resources, including three free books.
www.blochcancer.org

Cancer Care, Inc.—Information on specific cancers and clinical trials.
www.cancercare.org

Cancerfacts—A commercial site with information about various cancers and their treatments, as well as a guide to their cancer centers.
www.cancerfacts.com

CancerGuide—Provides a helpful 'tour' about obtaining information about cancer, including clinical trials.
www.cancerguide.org

CancerHelp UK—Information from The CRC Institute for Cancer Studies at The Medical School, The University of Birmingham, U.K.
www.medweb.bham.ac.uk/cancerhelp

CancerNet—An information service provided by the National Cancer Institute (NCI) or NIH.
www.cancernet.nci.nih.gov

CanSearch—A guide to cancer resources maintained by the National Coalition for Cancer Survivorship.
www.cansearch.org

Choice In Dying—Advocates recognition and protection of individual rights at the end of life.
www.choices.org

Commonweal—A health and environmental research institute with several programs including a one-week cancer residency retreat.
www.commonweal.org

ECaP—Exceptional Cancer Patients—Bernie Siegel's speaking schedule; resource materials; training opportunities.
www.ecap-online.org

Emphysema Foundation—Basic site on emphysema.
www.emphysema.net

Emphysema/Webfanatix—This site carries much information on emphysema.
www.webfanatix.com/emphysema...resources.htm

HealingWell—A general source of information on diseases, disorders and chronic illness.
www.healingwell.com

Health-Center—A commercial site with information on 400 health topics.
www.health-center.com

Healthfinder—A service of the U.S. Department of Health and Human Services with information on and links to many health-related subjects.
www.healthfinder.gov

Health Insurance Association of America (HIAA)—Publishes a free pamphlet on health insurance. Website answers many questions.
www.hiaa.org

Health Insurance Counseling and Advocacy Program (HICAP)—A national Medicare assistance program for the elderly and disabled.
www.csuchico.edu/mssp/HICAP.html

HealthWeb—Developed under contract with the National Library of Medicine and contains information on a large variety of health-related subjects.
www.healthweb.org

HealthyLives—A commercial source by GlaxoSmithKline with detailed information on many diseases.
www.healthylives.com

The Hemlock Society—Information on options for a peaceful death.
www.hemlock.org

HIV/AIDS—This is the American Medical Association site on HIV/AIDS with lots of information and resources.
www.ama-assn.org/insight/spec...con/hiv...aids/supptgrp.htm

HIVCyberMall—A general site for HIV/AIDS with many categories and links.
www.hivcybermall.org/homepage.htm

IBIS—An informational link to many resources maintained by the Integrative Medical Arts Group, Inc.
www.healthwwweb.com

Links to Cancer Institutes and Research Centers—Information about specific cancers as well as message boards and links to support groups.
www.seidata.com/~marriage/rcancer.html

Mayo Clinic—This site is specifically for their Heart Center, with information on diseases of the heart plus links to other heart health organizations.
www.mayohealth.org/mayo/common/htm/heartpg.htm

Medicaid—The U.S. government's Medicaid website.
www.hcfa.gov/medicaid/medicaid.htm

Medicare—The U.S. government's Medicare website.
www.medicare.gov

MEDLINE—This is the National Library of Medicine's premier bibliographic database.
www.nlm.nih.gov/databases/medline.html

Merck—This gives you free access to the complete *The Merck Manual*, the most widely used general medical text.
www. merck.com

National Alliance of Breast Cancer Organizations (NABCO)—A network of over 400 organizations dealing with breast cancer. Good information.
www.nabco.org

National Association of Community Health Centers Inc.—Provides a listing of local, nonprofit, community-owned health care programs serving low income and medically underserved urban and rural communities.
www.nachc.com

National Cancer Institute (NCI)—This website connects you to all of NCI's services.
www.nci.nih.gov

National Center for Complementary and Alternative Medicine (NCCAM)—This center supports basic and applied research and training, and disseminates information on complementary and alternative medicine to practitioners and the public.
www.altmed.od.nih.gov

National Foundation for Alternative Medicine—Collects and reports information worldwide on medical alternatives.
www.nfam.org

National Heart Foundation—The website of the American Health Assistance Foundation with much information on heart diseases.
www.ahaf.org/hrtstrok/about/hsabout...body.htm

National Hospice Organization (NHO)—Information about hospices and where to find them.
www.nho.org

National Institutes of Health (NIH)—The U.S. government's central research agency on health matters.
www.nih.gov

National Kidney Foundation—Basic access to information and resources on kidney diseases.
www.kidney.org/patients

Neuromuscular Disease Center—Information on various neuro-muscular diseases.
www.neuro.wustl.edu/neuromuscular

Nutrition Navigator—The Tufts University website for those who seek reliable information on nutrition.
www.navigator.tufts.edu

Office of Dietary Supplements (ODS)—They maintain an international bibliographic database on information on dietary supplements.
www.odp.od.nih.gov/ods/databases/databases.html

OncoLink—University of Pennsylvania Cancer Center—This is a superb website with up-to-date information in many categories to help cancer patients. Some of the information is available in Spanish.
www.oncolink.upenn.edu

Patient Advocate Foundation—Provides education and legal counseling about managed care, insurance, and financial issues for cancer patients.
www.patientadvocate.org

Simonton Cancer Center—Information about Dr. O. Carl Simonton's programs.
www.lainet.com/~simonton

Toxicology Data Network (TOXNET)—Databases on toxicology, hazardous chemicals and related areas.
www.toxnet.nlm.nih.gov/servlets/toxnet.pages.homepage

Veris Resource Information Service—A particularly good source for information on antioxidants.
www.veris-online.org

Veterans Administration—Health services for American veterans.
www.va.gov

Useful Phone Numbers

The following are some useful phone numbers in alphabetical order:

American Cancer Society: 800-227-2345

American Pain Society: 847-375-4700

American Society of Clinical Hypnosis: 847-297-3317

Association of Oncology Social Work: 410-614-3990

R.A. Bloch Cancer Foundation: 800-433-0464

Cancer Care, Inc.: 800-813-4673

CancerFax: 301-402-5874

Cancer Information Service (CIS): 800-422-6237

Choice In Dying: 800-989-WILL

Exceptional Cancer Patients (ECaP): 814-337-8192

Health Insurance Association of America (HIAA): 202-824-1600

Health Insurance Counseling and Advocacy Program (HICAP): 800-822-0109

Medicare: 800-633-4227

Make Today Count: 800-432-2273

Milton H. Erickson Foundation: 602-956-6196

National Association of Community Health Centers Inc.: 202-659-8008

National Cancer Institute: 800-422-6237

National Coalition for Cancer Survivorship: 888-650-9127

National Family Caregivers Association: 800-896-3650

National Hospice Organization: 800-658-8898

Needy Meds: 334-662-0023

Oncology Nursing Society: 412-921-7373

Patient Advocate Foundation: 800-532-5274

Veterans Administration: 800-827-1000

Wellness Community: 888-793-WELL

Y-Me: 800-221-2141

Appendix C

Patient's Bill of Rights

Bernie Siegel (1986, pp. 127–128) gives the following as a patient's bill of rights. It is written as an open letter to physicians.

Dear Doctor:

Please don't conceal the diagnosis. We both know I came to you to learn if I have cancer or some other serious disease. If I know what I have, I know what I am fighting, and there is less to fear. If you hide the name and the facts, you deprive me of the chance to help myself. When you are questioning whether I should be told, I already know. You may feel better if you don't tell me, but your deception hurts.

Do not tell me how long I have to live! I alone can decide how long I will live. It is my desires, my goals, my values, my strengths, and my will to live that will make the decision.

Teach me and my family about how and why my illness happened to me. Help me and my family to live *now*. Tell me about nutrition and my body's needs. Tell me how to handle the knowledge and how my mind and body can work together. Healing comes from within, but I want to combine my strength with yours. If you and I are a team, I will live a longer and better life.

Doctor, don't let your negative beliefs, your fears, and your prejudices affect my health. Don't stand in the way of my getting well and exceeding your expectations. Give me the chance to be the exception to your statistics.

Teach me about your beliefs and therapies and help me to incorporate them into mine. However, remember that my beliefs are the most important. What I don't believe in won't help me.

You must learn what my disease means to me—death, pain, or fear of the unknown. If my belief system accepts alternative therapy and not recognized therapy, do not desert me. Please try to convert to my beliefs, and be patient and await my conversion. It may come at a time when I am desperately ill and in great need of your therapy.

Doctor, teach me and my family to live with my problem when I am not with you. Take time for our questions and give us your attention when we need it. It is important that I feel free to talk with you and question you. I will live a longer and more meaningful life if you and I can develop a significant relationship. I need you in my life to achieve my new goals.

Appendix D

The Wellness Community Patient/Oncologist Statement

The effective treatment of serious illness requires considerable effort by both the patient and the physician. A clear understanding by both of us as to what each of us can realistically and reasonably expect of the other will do much to enhance the outlook. I am giving this 'statement' to you as one step in making our relationship as effective and productive as possible. It might be helpful if you would read this statement and, if you think it appropriate, discuss it with me. *As your physician I will make every effort to*:

1. Provide you with the care most likely to be beneficial to you.
2. Inform and educate you about your situation, and the various treatment alternatives. How detailed an explanation is given will be dependent upon your specific desires.
3. Encourage you to ask questions about your illness and its treatment, and answer your questions as clearly as possible. I will attempt to answer the questions asked by your family; however, my primary responsibility is to you, and I will discuss your medical situation only with those people authorized by you.
4. Remain aware that all major decisions about the course of your care will be made by you. However, I will accept the responsibility for making certain decisions if you want me to.
5. Assist you to obtain other professional opinions if you desire, or if I believe it to be in your best interest.
6. Relate to you as one competent adult to another, always attempting to consider your emotional, social, and psychological needs as well as your physical needs.
7. Spend a reasonable amount of time with you on each return visit unless required by something urgent to do otherwise, and give you my undivided attention during that time.
8. Honor all appointment times unless required by something urgent to do otherwise.

9. Return phone calls as promptly as possible, especially those you indicate are urgent.
10. Make test results available promptly if you desire such reports.
11. Provide you with any information you request concerning my professional training, experience, philosophy and fees.
12. Respect your desire to try treatments that might not be conventionally accepted. However, I will give you my honest opinion about such unconventional treatments.
13. Maintain my active support and attention throughout the course of the illness.

I hope that you as the patient will make every effort to:

1. Comply with our agreed-upon treatment plan.
2. Be as candid as possible with me about what you need and expect from me.
3. Inform me if you desire another professional opinion.
4. Inform me of all forms of therapy you are involved with.
5. Honor all appointment times unless required by something urgent to do otherwise.
6. Be as considerate as possible of my need to adhere to a schedule to see other patients.
7. Make all phone calls to me during the working hours. Call on nights and weekends only when absolutely necessary.
8. Coordinate the requests of your family and confidants, so that I do not have to answer the same questions about you to several different persons.

Taken from Benjamin (1995, pp. 210–212).

Appendix E

Living Will Declaration (State of Ohio)

I, _____, presently residing at _____, Ohio, (the 'Declarant'), being of sound mind and not under or subject to any duress, fraud or undue influence, intending to create a Living Will Declaration under Chapter 2133 of the Ohio Revised Code, as amended from time to time, do voluntarily make known my desire that my dying shall not be artificially prolonged. If I am unable to give directions regarding the use of life-sustaining treatment when I am in a terminal condition or a permanently unconscious state, it is my intention that the Living Will Declaration shall be honored by my family and physicians as the final expression of my legal right to refuse medical or surgical treatment. I am a competent adult who understands and accepts the consequences of such refusal and the purpose and effect of this document.

In the event I am in a terminal condition, I do hereby declare and direct that my attending physician shall:

1. administer no life-sustaining treatment;
2. withdraw such treatment if such treatment has commenced; and
3. permit me to die naturally and provide me with only that care necessary to make me comfortable and to relieve my pain but not to postpone my death.

In the event that I am in a permanently unconscious state, I do hereby declare and direct that my attending physician shall:

1. administer no life-sustaining treatment, except for the provision of artificially or technologically supplied nutrition or hydration, unless in the following paragraph, I have authorized its withholding or withdrawal;
2. withdraw such treatment if such treatment has commenced; and
3. permit me to die naturally and provide me with only that care necessary to make me comfortable and to relieve my pain but not to postpone my death.

❑ _____ IN ADDITION, IF I HAVE MARKED THE FORE-GOING BOX AND HAVE PLACED MY INITIALS ON THE LINE ADJACENT TO IT, I AUTHORIZE MY ATTENDING PHYSICIAN TO WITHHOLD, OR IN THE EVENT THAT TREATMENT HAS ALREADY COMMENCED, TO WITHDRAW, THE PROVISION OF ARTIFICIALLY OR TECHNOLOGICALLY SUPPLIED NUTRI-TION AND HYDRATION, IF I AM IN A PERMANENTLY UNCONSCIOUS STATE AND IF MY ATTENDING PHYSICIAN AND AT LEAST ONE OTHER PHYSICIAN WHO HAS EXAM-INED ME DETERMINE, TO A REASONABLE DEGREE OF MEDI-CAL CERTAINTY AND IN ACCORDANCE WITH REASONABLE MEDICAL STANDARDS, THAT SUCH NUTRITION OR HYDRA-TION WILL NOT OR NO LONGER WILL SERVE TO PROVIDE COMFORT TO ME OR ALLEVIATE MY PAIN.

In the event my attending physician determines that life-sustaining treatment should be withheld or withdrawn, he or she shall make a good faith effort and use reasonable diligence to notify one of the persons named below in the following order of priority:

1. (Name) _____, (Relationship) _____
presently residing at (Address) _____
_____, Phone _____

2. (Name) _____, (Relationship) _____
presently residing at (Address) _____,
_____Phone _____

For the purposes of this Living Will Declaration:

(A)   'Life-sustaining treatment' means any medical procedure, treatment, intervention, or other measure including artifi-cially or technologically supplied nutrition and hydration that, when administered, will serve principally to prolong the process of dying.

(B)   'TERMINAL CONDITION' MEANS AN IRREVERSIBLE, INCURABLE, AND UNTREATABLE CONDITION CAUSED BY DISEASE, ILLNESS, OR INJURY TO WHICH, TO A REASONABLE DEGREE OF MEDICAL CERTAINTY AS DETERMINED IN ACCORDANCE

WITH REASONABLE MEDICAL STANDARDS BY MY ATTENDING PHYSICIAN AND ONE OTHER PHYSICIAN WHO HAS EXAMINED ME, BOTH OF THE FOLLOWING APPLY:

(1)   THERE CAN BE NO RECOVERY, AND

(2)   DEATH IS LIKELY TO OCCUR WITHIN A RELATIVELY SHORT TIME IF LIFE-SUSTAINING TREATMENT IS NOT ADMINISTERED.

(C)   'PERMANENTLY UNCONSCIOUS STATE' MEANS A STATE OF PERMANENT UNCONSCIOUSNESS THAT, TO A REASONABLE DEGREE OF MEDICAL CERTAINTY AS DETERMINED IN ACCORDANCE WITH REASONABLE MEDICAL STANDARDS BY MY ATTENDING PHYSICIAN AND ONE OTHER PHYSICIAN WHO HAS EXAMINED ME, IS CHARACTERIZED BY BOTH OF THE FOLLOWING:

(1)   I AM IRREVERSIBLY UNAWARE OF MYSELF AND MY ENVIRONMENT, AND

(2)   THERE IS A TOTAL LOSS OF CEREBRAL CORTICAL FUNCTIONING, RESULTING IN MY HAVING NO CAPACITY TO EXPERIENCE PAIN OR SUFFERING.

(D)   [Note: The author (RB) added this section and the following medical directive.] The attached Medical Directive gives specific details of my wishes for four separate situations for additional guidance. _____ (initials)

I understand the purpose and effect of this document and sign my name to this Living Will Declaration after careful deliberation on (Date) _____ at (City) _____, Ohio.

(Declarant's signature) _____

THIS LIVING WILL DECLARATION WILL NOT BE VALID UNLESS IT IS EITHER (1) SIGNED BY TWO ELIGIBLE

WITNESSES AS DEFINED BELOW WHO ARE PRESENT WHEN YOU SIGN OR ACKNOWLEDGE YOUR SIGNATURE OR (2) ACKNOWLEDGED BEFORE A NOTARY PUBLIC.

I attest that the Declarant signed or acknowledged this Living Will Declaration in my presence, and that the Declarant appears to be of sound mind and not under or subject to any duress, fraud or undue influence. I further attest that I am not the attending physician of the Declarant, I am not the administrator of a nursing home in which the Declarant is receiving care, and that I am an adult not related to the Declarant by blood, marriage or adoption.

Signature: _____   Residence Address: _____

Print Name: _____   _____

_____   _____

Date: _____   _____

Signature: _____   Residence Address: _____

Print Name: _____   _____

_____   _____

Date: _____   _____

(OR CERTIFICATION BY A NOTARY PUBLIC.)

[NOTE: This document was prepared and distributed by the Ohio State Bar Association and their preparation of the document is gratefully acknowledged.]

* * * * * * * * * * * * * *

The following is a detailed **medical directive** that adds some specific directions to the preceding Living Will Declaration. There are four separate situations described and for each of these there are 12 interventions described. For a few choices, 'NA' means 'Not Applicable.' Due to space considerations only *one* column of four choices is provided—you would actually have to fill out four such columns, i.e., one for each situation. After the introductory material for the medical directive, each of the four situations is given in detail, then the table.

My Medical Directive

This Medical Directive expresses, and shall stand for, my wishes regarding medical treatments in the event that illness should make me unable to communicate them directly. I make this Directive being 18 years or more of age, of sound mind, and appreciating the consequences of my decisions.

SITUATION A: If I am in a coma or a persistent vegetative state and, in the opinion of my physician and several consultants, have no hope of regaining awareness and higher mental functions no matter what is done, then my wishes regarding the use of the following, if considered medically reasonable, would be:

SITUATION B: If I am in a coma and, in the opinion of my physician and several consultants, have a small likelihood of recovering fully, a slightly larger likelihood of surviving with permanent brain damage, and a much larger likelihood of dying, then my wishes regarding use of the following, if considered medically reasonable, would be:

SITUATION C: If I have brain damage or some brain disease that in the opinion of my physician and several consultants cannot be reversed and that makes me unable to recognize people or to speak understandably, and I also have a terminal illness, such as incurable cancer, that will likely be the cause of my death, then my wishes regarding the use of the following, if considered medically reasonable, would be:

SITUATION D: If I have brain damage or some brain disease that in the opinion of my physician and several consultants cannot be reversed and that makes me unable to recognize people or to speak understandably, but I have no terminal illness, and I can live in this condition for a long time, then my wishes regarding use of the following, if considered medically reasonable, would be:

Type of Intervention	Situation A — I want	B — I want treatment tried. If no clear improvement, stop	C — I am undecided	D — I do not want
Cardiopulmonary Resuscitation: if at point of death, using drugs and electric shock to keep the heart beating; artificial breathing.		NA		
Mechanical Breathing: breathing by machine.				
Artificial Nutrition and Hydration: giving nutrition and fluid through a tube in the veins, nose, or stomach.				
Major Surgery: such as removing the gall bladder or part of the intestines.		N/A		
Kidney Dialysis: cleaning the blood by machine or by part of the intestines.				
Chemotherapy: using drugs to fight cancer.				
Minor Surgery: such as removing some tissue from an infected toe.		N/A		
Invasive Diagnostic Tests: such as using a flexible tube to look into the stomach.		N/A		
Blood or Blood Products: such as giving transfusions. **Antibiotics:** using drugs to fight infection.				
Simple Diagnostic Tests: such as performing blood tests or x-rays.		N/A		
Pain Medications, even if they dull consciousness and directly shorten my life.				

(The author's choices were "I do not want" for all interventions except pain medications where he checked "I want.")

In addition to the above, this Medical Directive includes a section on organ donation, as follows:

ORGAN DONATION
I hereby make this anatomical gift to take effect upon my death. (please check boxes and fill in where appropriate.)

I give: ❑ my body ❑ any needed organs or parts
❑ the following organs or parts _____
to: ❑ the following person or institution _____

❑ the physician in attendance at my death
❑ the hospital in which I die
❑ the following named physician, hospital, storage bank, or other medical institution: _____
for the following purposes:

❑ any purpose authorized by law
❑ transplantation ❑ therapy of another person
❑ research ❑ medical education

MY PERSONAL STATEMENT
(Add details here on anything else you wish using additional space as needed.) _____
_____

Name (printed) _____

Name (signed) _____

Witness 1 (signed) _____

Witness 2 (signed) _____

Date _____

[Please note that each individual state in the U.S. and each country will have its own legal standards about these matters.]

Appendix F

Christian Affirmation of Life

To my family, friends, physician, lawyer, and clergyman:

I believe that each individual person is created by God our Father in love and that God retains a loving relationship to each person throughout human life and eternity.

I believe that Jesus Christ lived, suffered, and died for me and that his suffering, death, and resurrection prefigured and made possible the death-resurrection process which I now anticipate.

I believe that each person's worth and dignity derives from the relationship of love that God has for each individual person and not from one's usefulness or effectiveness in society.

I believe that God our Father has entrusted me a shared dominion with him over my earthly existence so that I am bound to use ordinary means to preserve my life but I am free to refuse extraordinary means to prolong my life.

I believe that through death life is not taken away but merely changed, and though I may experience fear, suffering, and sorrow, by the grace of the Holy Spirit, I hope to accept death as a free human act which enables me to surrender this life and to be united with God for eternity.

Because of my belief:

I request that I be informed as death approaches so that I may continue to prepare for the full encounter with Christ through the help of the sacraments and the consolation and prayers of my family and friends.

I request that, if possible, I be consulted concerning the medical procedures which might be used to prolong my life as death approaches. If I can no longer take part in decisions concerning my own future and if there is no reasonable expectation of my recovery from physical and mental disability, I request that no extraordinary means be used to prolong my life.

I request, though I wish to join my suffering to the suffering of Jesus so I may be united fully with him in the act of death-resurrection, that my pain, if unbearable, be alleviated. However, no means should be used with the intention of shortening my life.

I request, because I am a sinner and in need of reconciliation and because my faith, hope, and love may not overcome all fear and doubt, that my family, friends, and the whole Christian community join me in prayer and mortification as I prepare for the great personal act of dying.

Finally, I request that after my death, my family, friends, and the whole Christian community pray for me, and rejoice with me because of the mercy and love of the Trinity, with whom I hope to be united for all eternity.

Signed _____ Date _____

Note: This document was approved by the Board of Trustees of The Catholic Hospital Association.

Appendix G

The Christian Living Will

To My Family, Physician, Clergy, Attorney, and Medical Facility:

First: I, _____, as a Christian, believe that "Whether we live or whether we die, we are the Lord's" (Romans 14:8). If death is certain, so is the faithfulness of God in death as in life. With this high hope to sustain me, I wish to be responsible in dying as well as in living.

Second: To this end, I implore all those responsible for my care and knowledgeable of my condition to be completely honest with me in the event of a terminal illness, so that I may make my own decisions and preparations as much as possible.

Third: If there is no reasonable expectation of my recovery and I am no longer able to share decisions concerning my future, I ask that I be allowed to die and not be kept alive indefinitely by artificial means or heroic measures. I ask that drugs be administered to me as needed to relieve terminal suffering even if this may hasten the moment of my death. I am not asking that my life be directly taken, but that my dying be not unreasonably prolonged if my condition is hopeless, my deterioration irreversible, and the maintenance of my life an overwhelming responsibility for my family or an unfair monopoly of medical resources.

Fourth: This request is made thoughtfully while I am in good health and spirits. Even if this document be not binding legally, I beg those who care for me to honor its intent, which is in part to relieve them of some of the burden of this decision. In this way, I take responsibility for my own death and gladly give my life back to God.

Date: _____ Signed: _____

Witness: _____

Coping

Reaffirmations:

Date: _____ Signed: _____

Copies given to: _____

Appendix H

Durable Power of Attorney for Health Care (Ohio)

1. DESIGNATION OF ATTORNEY-IN-FACT.
I, _____, presently residing at _____, Ohio, (the 'Principal') being of sound mind and not under or subject to duress, fraud or undue influence, intending to create a Durable Power of Attorney for Health Care under Chapter 1337 of the Ohio Revised Code, as amended from time to time, do hereby, designate and appoint:

(Name) _____

(Relationship) _____ presently residing at _____

Phone _____ as my attorney-in-fact who shall act as my agent to make health care decisions for me as authorized in this document.

2. GENERAL STATEMENT OF AUTHORITY GRANTED.
I hereby grant to my agent full power and authority to make all health care decisions for me to the same extent that I could make such decisions for myself if I had the capacity to do so, at any time during which I do not have the capacity to make informed decisions for myself. Such agent shall have the authority to give, to withdraw or to refuse to give informed consent to any medical and nursing procedure, treatment, intervention or other measure used to maintain, diagnose or treat my physical or mental condition. In exercising this authority, my agent shall make health care decisions that are consistent with my desires as stated in this document or otherwise made known to my agent by me or, if I have not made my desires known, that are, in the judgment of my agent, in my best interests.

3. ADDITIONAL AUTHORITIES OF AGENT.
Where necessary or desirable to implement health care decisions that my agent is authorized to make pursuant to this document, my

agent has the power and the authority to do any and all of the following:

(a) If I am in a terminal condition, to withdraw or to refuse to give informed consent to life-sustaining treatment, including the provision of artificially or technologically supplied nutrition or hydration;
(b) If I am in a permanently unconscious state, to give, to withdraw or to refuse to give informed consent to life-sustaining treatment; provided, however, my agent is not authorized to refuse or direct the withdrawal of artificially or technologically supplied nutrition or hydration unless I have specifically authorized such refusal or withdrawal in Paragraph 4;
(c) To request, review, and receive any information, verbal or written, regarding my physical or mental health, including, but not limited to, all of my medical and health care facility records;
(d) To execute on my behalf any releases or other documents that may be required in order to obtain this information;
(e) To consent to the further disclosure of this information if necessary;
(f) To select, employ, and discharge health care personnel, such as physicians, nurses, therapists and other medical professionals, including individuals and services providing home health care, as my agent shall determine to be appropriate;
(g) To select and contract with any medical or health care facility on my behalf, including, but not limited to, hospitals, nursing homes, assisted residence facilities, and the like; and
(h) To execute on my behalf any or all of the following:
(1) Documents that are written consents to medical treatment, Do Not Resuscitate orders, or similar other orders;
(2) Documents that are written requests that I be transferred to another facility, written requests to be discharged against medical advice, or other similar requests; and
(3) Any other document necessary or desirable to implement health care decisions that my agent is authorized to make pursuant to this document.

4. WITHDRAWAL OF NUTRITION AND HYDRATION WHEN IN A PERMANENTLY UNCONSCIOUS STATE.

❏ _____ IF I HAVE MARKED THE FOREGOING BOX AND HAVE PLACED MY INITIALS ON THE LINE ADJACENT TO IT,

MY AGENT MAY REFUSE, OR IN THE EVENT TREATMENT HAS ALREADY COMMENCED, WITHDRAW INFORMED CONSENT TO THE PROVISION OF ARTIFICIALLY OR TECHNOLOGICALLY SUPPLIED NUTRITION AND HYDRATION IF I AM IN A PERMANENTLY UNCONSCIOUS STATE AND IF MY ATTENDING PHYSICIAN AND AT LEAST ONE OTHER PHYSICIAN WHO HAS EXAMINED ME DETERMINE, TO A REASONABLE DEGREE OF MEDICAL CERTAINTY AND IN ACCORDANCE WITH REASONABLE MEDICAL STANDARDS, THAT SUCH NUTRITION OR HYDRATION WILL NOT OR NO LONGER WILL SERVE TO PROVIDE COMFORT TO ME OR ALLEVIATE MY PAIN.

5. DESIGNATION OF ALTERNATE AGENT.
Because I wish that an agent shall be available to exercise the authorities granted hereunder at all times, I further designate each of the following individuals to succeed to such authorities and to serve under this instrument, in the order named, if at any time the agent first named (or any alternate designee) is not readily available or is unwilling to serve or to continue to serve:

First Alternate Agent: (Name) _____
(Relationship) _____
presently residing at _____ Phone: _____

Second Alternate Agent: (Name) _____
(Relationship) _____
presently residing at _____ Phone: _____

Each alternate shall have and exercise all of the authority conferred above.

6. NO EXPIRATION DATE.
This Durable Power of Attorney for Health Care shall not be affected by my disability or by lapse of time. This Durable Power of Attorney for Health Care shall have no expiration date.

7. SEVERABILITY.
Any invalid or unenforceable power, authority or provision of this instrument shall not affect another power, authority or provision or the appointment of my agent to make health care decisions.

8. PRIOR DESIGNATIONS REVOKED.

I hereby revoke any prior Durable Power of Attorney for Health Care executed by me under Chapter 1337 of the Ohio Revised Code.

I understand the purpose and effect of this document and sign my name to this Durable Power of Attorney for Health Care after careful deliberation on (Date) _____ at (City) _____, Ohio.

(Signature of Principal) _____

THIS DURABLE POWER OF ATTORNEY FOR HEALTH CARE WILL NOT BE VALID UNLESS IT IS EITHER (1) SIGNED BY TWO ELIGIBLE WITNESSES AS DEFINED BELOW WHO ARE PRESENT WHEN YOU SIGN OR ACKNOWLEDGE YOUR SIGNATURE OR (2) ACKNOWLEDGED BEFORE A NOTARY PUBLIC.

I attest that the principal signed or acknowledged this Durable Power of Attorney for Health Care in my presence, that the principal appears to be of sound mind and not under or subject to duress, fraud, or undue influence. I further attest that I am not the agent designated in this document, I am not the attending physician of the principal, I am not the administrator of a nursing home in which the principal is receiving care, and I am an adult not related to the principal by blood, marriage or adoption.

Signature: _____

Residence Address: _____

Print Name: _____

Date: _____

Signature: _____

Residence Address: _____

Print Name: _____

Date: _____

OR ACKNOWLEDGMENT BY A NOTARY PUBLIC.

[NOTE: This document was prepared and is distributed by the Ohio State Bar Association, and we gratefully acknowledge their work on the document.]

References

Achterberg, J., Dossey, B., & Kolkmeier, L. (1994). *Rituals of healing: using imagery for health and wellness.* New York: Bantam Books.

Adams, P. (1998). *Gesundheit! Bringing good health to you, the medical system, and society through physician service, complementary therapies, humor, and joy.* Rochester, VT: Healing Arts Press.

Ahmad, N., & Mukhtar, H. (1999). Green tea polyphenols and cancer: Biological mechanisms and practical implication. *Nutrition Reviews 57* (3): 78–83.

Ames, B.N., Shigenaga, M.K., & Hagen, T.M. (1993). Oxidants, antioxidants, and the degenerative diseases of aging. *Proceedings of the National Academy of Science (USA) 90*: 7915–7922.

Andrews, C. (1997). *The circle of simplicity. Return to the good life.* New York: HarperCollins Publishers.

Bailey, C. (1991). *The new fit or fat.* Boston: Houghton Mifflin Company.

Balentine, D.A., Albano, M.C., & Nair, M.G. (1999). Role of medicinal plants, herbs, and spices in protecting human health. *Nutrition Reviews 57* (9, II): S41–S45.

Bank, W.O. (1985). Hypnotic suggestion for the control of bleeding in the angiography suite. In S.R. Lankton (Ed.), *Ericksonian Monographs* No. 1. *Elements and dimensions of an Ericksonian Approach.* (pp. 76–88). New York: Brunner/Mazel.

Battino, R. (2000). *Guided imagery and other approaches to healing.* Bancyfelin, Carmarthen, UK: Crown House Publishing Ltd.

Battino, R., & South, T.L. (1999). *Ericksonian approaches: A comprehensive manual.* Bancyfelin, Carmarthen, UK: Crown House Publishing Ltd.

Benjamin, H.H. (1995). *The Wellness Community guide to fighting and recovery from cancer.* New York: Jeremy P. Tarcher/Putnam Books.

Benson, H. (1975). *The relaxation response.* New York: William Morrow and Co.

Benson, H. (1984). *Beyond the relaxation response.* New York: Times Books.

Benson, H. (With Stark, M.). (1996). *Timeless healing—the power and biology of belief.* New York: Scribner.

Bloch, A.S. (Ed.) (1990). *Nutrition management of the cancer patient.* Rockville, MD: Aspen Publishers Inc.

Bloch, A.S. (1994). Feeding the cancer patient: Where have we come from, where are we going? *Nutrition in Clinical Practice 9*: 87–89.

Bloch, A.S. (2000). *Oncology, diet, & nutrition. Patient education resource manual.* Rockville, MD: Aspen Publications Inc.

Brooks, A.M. (1985). *The grieving time: A year's account of recovery from loss.* Garden City, NY: The Dial Press (Doubleday & Co.).

Cheek, D.B. (1959). Unconscious perception of meaningful sounds during surgical anesthesia as revealed under hypnosis. *American Journal of Clinical Hypnosis 1*: 101–113.

Cheek, D.B. (1960a). Use of preoperative hypnosis to protect patients from careless conversation. *American Journal of Clinical Hypnosis 3*(2), 101–102.

Cheek, D.B. (1960b). What does the surgically anesthetized patient hear? *Rocky Mountain Medical Journal 57*, January: 49–53.

Cheek, D.B. (1961). Unconscious reactions and surgical risk. *Western Journal of Surgery, Obstetrics, and Gynecology 69*: 325–328.

Cheek, D.B. (1964). Further evidence of persistence of hearing under chem-anesthesia: detailed case report. *American Journal of Clinical Hypnosis 7*(1): 55–59.

Cheek, D.B. (1965). Can surgical patients react to what they hear under anesthesia? *Journal American Association Nurse Anesthetists 33*: 30–38.

Cheek, D.B. (1966). The meaning of continued hearing sense under general anesthesia. *American Journal of Clinical Hypnosis 8*: 275–280.

Cheek, D.B. (1981). Awareness of meaningful sounds under general anesthesia: considerations and a review of the literature. In H.J. Wain (Ed.), *Theoretical and clinical aspects of hypnosis.* Miami: Symposia Specialists Inc.

Cheek, D.B. (1994). *Hypnosis. The application of ideomotor techniques.* Needham Heights, MA: Allyn and Bacon.

Clark, L.C., Combs, G.F., Turnbull, B.W., Slate, E.H., Chalker, D.K., Chow, J., Davis, L.S., Glover, R.A., Graham, G.F., Gross, E.G., Krongrad, A., Lesher, J.L., Park, H.K., Sanders, B.B., Smith, C.L., & Taylor, J.R. (1996). Effect of selenium supplementation for cancer prevention in patients with carcinoma of the skin. *Journal of the American Medical Association 276* (24): 1957–1963.

Comstock, G.W., Bush, T.L., & Helzlsouer, K. (1992). Serum retinol, beta-carotene, vitamin E and selenium as related to subsequent cancer of specific sites. *American Journal of Epidemiology 135* (2): 115–121.

Connor, W.E., & Connor, S.L. (1989). Dietary treatment of familial hypercholesterolemia. *Arteriosclerosis (Suppl. 1) 9* (1): I91–I105.

Cooper, K.H. (1996). *Advanced nutritional therapies.* Nashville: Thomas Nelson, Publishers.

Cousins, N. (1979, 1981). *Anatomy of an illness.* New York: W.W. Norton & Co.

Cousins, N. (1984). *The healing heart.* New York: Bantam Books.

de Shazer, S. (1985). *Keys to solution in brief therapy.* New York: W.W. Norton & Co.

Doka, K.J. (1993). *Living with life-threatening illness. A guide for patients, their families, & caregivers.* San Francisco: Jossey-Bass Publishers.

Dossey, L. (1991). *Meaning & medicine. Lessons from a doctor's tales of breakthrough and healing.* New York: Bantam Books.

Dossey, L. (1993). *Healing words. The power of prayer and the practice of medicine.* New York: HarperCollins Publishers.

Dossey, L. (1996). *Prayer is good medicine.* New York: HarperCollins Publishers.

Dossey, L. (1997). *Be careful what you pray for ... you just might get it.* New York: HarperCollins Publishers.

Elgin, D. (1981). *Voluntary simplicity. Toward a way of life that is outwardly simple, inwardly rich.* New York: William Morrow and Company.

Esterling, B.A., L'Abate, L., Murray, E.J., & Pennebaker, J.W. (1999). Empirical foundations for writing in prevention and psychotherapy: Mental and physical health outcomes. *Clinical Psychology Review 19*: 79–96.

Evans, W., & Rosenberg, I.H. (1992). *Biomarkers. The 10 keys to prolonging vitality.* New York: Fireside (Simon & Schuster).

Fink, J.M. (1997). *Third opinion. An international directory to alternative therapy centers for the treatment and prevention of cancer and other degenerative diseases.* Garden City Park, NY: Avery Publishing Group.

Frankl, V.E. (1959; 1962, Rev. Ed.; 1984, 3rd Ed.). *Man's search for meaning.* New York: Simon and Schuster.

Gifford, K.D. (1998). The Mediterranean diet as a food guide: The problem of culture and history. *Nutrition Today 33* (6): 233–243.

Hammerschlag, C.A. (1988). *The dancing healers.* New York: Harper-Collins.

Hammerschlag, C.A. (1993). *The theft of the spirit*. New York: Simon & Schuster.

Hammerschlag, C.A., & Silverman, H.D. (1997). *Healing ceremonies*. New York: Perigree Books.

Hamilton, S. (1999). As quoted in *Coping*, May/June, pp. 9–10.

Heber, D., Blackburn, G.L., & Go, V.L.W. (Eds.). (1999). *Nutritional oncology*. New York: Academic Press.

Helzlsouer, K.J., Bloch, G., Blumberg, J., Diplock, A.T., Levine, M., Marnett, L.J., Schulplein, R.J., Spence, J.T., & Simic, M.G. (1994). Summary of the roundtable discussion on strategies for cancer prevention: Diet, food, additives, supplements, and drugs. *Cancer Research (Suppl) 54:* 2044s–2051s.

Jacobson, E. (1938). *Progressive relaxation*. Chicago: University of Chicago Press.

Johnston, C.S. (1999). Biomarkers for establishing a tolerable upper intake level for vitamin C. *Nutrition Reviews 57*: 71–77.

Kim, Y.I. (1999). Folate and cancer prevention: A new medical application of folate beyond hyperhomocysteinemia and neural tube defects. *Nutrition Reviews 57* (10): 314–321.

Kirby, P. (2000). Real-world examples. Cancer treatment programs after massage. *Massage*. March/April. pp. 80–81.

Klein, S., & Koretz, R.L. (1994). Nutrition support in patients with cancer: What do the data really show? *Nutrition in Clinical Practice 9*: 91–100.

Koo, L.C. (1997). Diet and lung cancer 20+ years later: More questions than answers? *International Journal of Cancer Suppl 10*: 22–29.

L'Abate, L. (1992). *Programmed writing: A self-administered approach for interventions with individuals, couples, and families*. Pacific Grove, CA: Brooks/Cole.

L'Abate, L. (1997). Distance writing and computer-assisted training. In S.R. Sauber (Ed.), *Managed mental health care: Major diagnostic and treatment approaches*. (pp. 133–163). Bristol, PA: Brunner/Mazel.

Lawlis, G.F. (1996). *Transpersonal medicine. A new approach to healing body-mind-spirit*. Boston: Shambhala.

Lazarou, J., Pomeranz, B.H., & Corey, P.N. (1998). Incidence of adverse drug reactions in hospitalized patients. A meta-analysis of prospective studies. *Journal of the American Medical Association, 279* (15): 1200–1205.

Lerner, M. (1996). *Choices in healing*. Cambridge, MA: The MIT Press.

LeShan, L. (1974). *How to meditate. A guide to self-discovery.* New York: Bantam Books.

LeShan, L. (1989). *Cancer as a turning point.* New York: Plume Books (Penguin Books).

Letters to the Editor. (1989). Psychological support for cancer patients. *The Lancet*, Nov. 18: 1209–1210; rebuttal letter, ibid., Dec. 16: p. 1447.

Levine, M. (1999). From molecules to menus: Recommendations for vitamin C intake. *Journal of the American College of Nutrition 18* (5): 524.

Linden, W. (1990). *Autogenic training. A clinical guide.* New York: The Guildford Press.

Luhrs, J. (1997). *The simple living guide.* New York: Broadway Books.

MacDonald, G. (2000). Easing the chemotherapy experience with massage. *Massage.* March/April. pp. 85–91.

Matarese, L., & Gottschlich, M.M. (eds.). (1998). *Contemporary nutrition support practice: A clinical guide.* Philadelphia: W.B. Saunders Company.

Meichenbaum, D., & Turk, D.C. (1987). *Facilitating treatment adherence: A practitioner's guidebook.* New York: Plenum Press.

Melzack, R., Stillwell, D.M., & Fox, E.J. (1977). Trigger points and acupuncture points for pain: correlations and implications. *Pain* 3: 3–23.

Melzack, R. (1990). The tragedy of needless pain. *Scientific American* 262: 27–33. Feb.

Meyer, M., & Kaplan, K.O. (1998). Good planning. *Choices. The Newsletter of Choices in Dying.* Vol. 7. No. 2. Summer 1998, pp. 1, 4–5.

Milstein, L.B. (1994). *Giving comfort. What you can do when someone you love is ill.* New York: Penguin Books.

Naparstek, B. (1994). *Staying well with guided imagery.* New York: Warner Books.

Ornish, D. (1991). *Dr. Dean Ornish's program for reversing heart disease.* New York: Ballantine Books.

Ottery, F.D. (1994). Rethinking nutritional support of the cancer patient: The new field of nutritional oncology. *Seminars in Oncology 21* (6): 770–778.

Pauling, L. (1976). *Vitamin C, the common cold and the flu.* San Francisco: W.H. Freeman and Co.

Pearson, R.E. (1961). Response to suggestions given under general anesthesia. *American Journal of Clinical Hypnosis 4*: 106–114.

Pennebaker, J.W. (1997). *Opening up: The healing power of confiding in others*. New York: Guildford.

Pritikin, N. (1982). *28 days to a longer healthier life*. New York: Simon and Schuster.

Pritikin, N., & McGrady, Jr., P. (1979). *The Pritikin program for diet and exercise*. New York: Grosset and Dunlap.

Rainwater, J. (1979). *You're in charge! A guide to becoming your own therapist*. Los Angeles: Guild of Tutors.

Remen, R.N. (1994). *Wounded healers*. Mill Valley, CA: Wounded Healer Press (Commonweal).

Remen, R.N. (1996). *Kitchen table wisdom. Stories that heal*. New York: Riverhead Books.

Remen, R.N. (2000). *My grandfather's blessings. Stories of strength, refuge, and belonging*. New York: Riverhead Books.

Rossi, E.L., & Cheek, D.B. (1988). *Mind-body therapy. Ideodynamic healing in hypnosis*. New York: W.W. Norton & Co.

St. James, E. (1994). *Simplify your life. 100 ways to slow down and enjoy the things that really matter*. New York: Hyperion.

Seligman, P.A., Fink, R., & Massey-Seligman, E.J. (1998). Approach to the seriously ill or terminal cancer patient who has a poor appetite. *Seminars in Oncology 25* (2, Suppl 6): 33–34.

Sharp, A.W., & Terbay, S.H. (1997). *Gifts. Two hospice professionals reveal messages from those passing on*. Far Hills, NJ: New Horizon Press.

Sharp, S.J., & Pocock, S.J. (1997). Time trends in serum cholesterol before cancer death. *Epidemiology 8* (2): 132–136.

Siegel, B. (1986). *Love, medicine and miracles*. New York: Harper and Row.

Siegel, B. (1989). *Peace, love, and healing*. New York: Harper and Row.

Siegel, B. (1993). *How to live between office visits*. New York: HarperCollins Publishers.

Siegel, B.S. (1998). *Prescriptions for living. Inspirational lessons from a joyful, loving life*. New York: HarperCollins Publishers.

Spiegel, D. (1985). The use of hypnosis in controlling cancer pain. *CA: Cancer J. Clin., 35*: 221.

Spiegel, D., Bloom, J.R., Kraemer, H.C., & Gottheil, E. (1989). Effect of psychosocial treatment on survival of patients with metastatic breast cancer. *Lancet 2* (8668): 888–891 (Oct. 14). Also, by the same author and colleagues, see: Spiegel, D. (1992). Hypnosis and related techniques in pain management. *Hospice Journal 8* (1–2): 89–119; Kogon, M.M., Biswas, A., Pearl, D., Carlson,

R.W., & Spiegel, D. (1997 July 15). Effects of medical and psycho-therapeutic treatment on the survival of women with metastatic breast cancer. *Cancer 80* (2): 225–230; Spiegel, D. (1996 June). Cancer and depression. *British Journal of Psychiatry—Supplement. (30)*: 109–116.; Spiegel, D. (1995 July). Essentials of psychotherapeutic intervention for cancer patients. *Supportive Care in Cancer 3* (4): 252–256; Spiegel, D. (1994 Aug. 15). Health caring. Psychological support for patients with cancer. *Cancer 74* (4 Suppl). 1453–1457; Spiegel, D. (1997 Feb.). Psychosocial aspects of breast cancer treatment. *Seminars in Oncology 24* (1 Suppl 1): S1-36–S1-47; Spiegel, D., Sands, S., & Koopman, C. (1994 Nov. 1). Pain and depression in patients with cancer. *Cancer 74* (9): 2570–2578.

Steiner, M. (1999). Vitamin E, a modifier of platelet function: Rationale and use in cardiovascular and cerebrovascular disease. *Nutrition Reviews 57* (10): 306–309.

Suter, P.M., & Vetter, W. (1999). Alcohol and ischemic stroke. *Nutrition Reviews 57* (10): 310–314.

Suzuki, D.T. (1964). *An introduction to Zen Buddhism.* New York: Grove Press.

The alpha-tocopherol, beta-carotene cancer prevention study group. (1994). *The New England Journal of Medicine 330* (15): 1029–1035.

Trichopoulou, A., & Lagiou, P. (1997). Healthy traditional Mediterranean diet: An expression of culture, history, and lifestyle. *Nutrition Reviews 55* (11): 383–389.

Trichopoulou, A., Vasilopoulou, E., & Lagiou, A. (1999). Mediterranean diet and coronary heart disease: Are antioxidants critical? *Nutrition Reviews 57* (8): 253–255.

U.S. Congress Office of Technology Assessment. (1990). *Unconventional cancer therapies.* Washington: Government Printing Office.

Ursini, F., Tubaro, F., Rong, J., & Sevanian, A. (1999). Optimization of nutrition: Polyphenols and vascular protection. *Nutrition Reviews 57* (8): 241–249.

Visioli, F.P., & Galli, C. (1998). The effect of minor constituents of olive oil on cardiovascular disease: New findings. *Nutrition Reviews 56* (5): 142–147.

Weil, A. (1972). *The natural mind. A new way of looking at drugs and the higher consciousness.* Boston: Houghton Mifflin Company.

Weil, A. (1995). *Spontaneous healing. How to discover and enhance your body's natural ability to maintain and heal itself.* New York: Fawcett Columbine.

Weil, A. (1995). *Natural health, natural medicine.* Boston: Houghton Mifflin Company.

Weil, A. (1996). *Eight weeks to optimal healing power.* New York: Knopf.

Whitney, E.N., Cataldo, C.B., & Rolfes, S.R. (1998). *Understanding normal and clinical nutrition,* 5th Ed. Belmont, CA: West-Wadsworth Publishing Co.

Willett, W.C. (1994). Diet and health: What should we eat? *Science 264:* 532–537.

Williams, D. (2000). Touching cancer patients. Guidelines for massage therapists. *Massage.* March/April. pp. 74–79.

World Cancer Research Fund in association with American Institute for Cancer Research. (1997). *Food, nutrition and the prevention of cancer: A global perspective.* Washington, DC: World Cancer Research Fund/American Institute for Cancer Research.

Wortman, C.B., & Silver., R.C. (1989). The myths of coping with loss. *Journal of Consulting and Clinical Psychology 57:* 349–357.

Zureik, M., Courbon, D., & Ducimetiere, P. (1997). Decline in serum total cholesterol and the risk of death from cancer. *Epidemiology 8* (2): 137–143.

Index

Ericksonian Approaches
A Comprehensive Manual
Rubin Battino, M.S. & Thomas L. South, Ph.D.

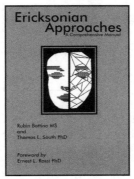

A highly acclaimed, outstanding training manual in the art of Ericksonian hypnotherapy. Accessible and elucidating, it provides a systematic approach to learning set against a clinical background, developing the reader's learning over twenty-two chapters which include: the history of hypnosis; myths and misconceptions; rapport-building skills; language forms; basic and advanced inductions; utilization of ideodynamic responses; basic and advanced metaphor and Ericksonian approaches in medicine, dentistry, substance abuse and life-challenging diseases.

CLOTH 564 PAGES ISBN: 1899836314

"This book should undoubtedly be read and re-read by any who consider themselves to be hypnotherapists. But it should not be limited to them. If people who are not interested in the subject of hypnotherapy are not drawn to it, this will be a loss for anyone who uses language in the course of therapeutic work ... I highly recommend this book."
—Barry Winbolt, *The New Therapist.*

Also available: a companion audiotape of Exercises and Demonstrations—ISBN 189983642X 65 mins.

Guided Imagery
and Other Approaches to Healing
Rubin Battino, M.S.

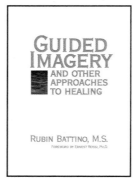

This book explores in detail the most powerful methods of healing. While focusing on *Guided Imagery*, a healing technique that fully exploits the connection between mind and body, it also extends its analysis to other healing techniques, including psychotherapy-based methods and alternative therapies, encouraging a multi-modal approach to healing. An essentially practical and accessible healing manual, *Guided Imagery* presents a breakdown of published guided imagery scripts, while investigating the language used in guided imagery, the skills required in rapport-building, and the most effective methods in inducing a state of relaxation. Pioneering new bonding and fusion healing methods, *Guided Imagery* also incorporates a useful section on preparing patients for surgery, and a chapter on Nutrition and Healing, by nutrition expert H. Ira Fritz, Ph.D., plus a chapter on Native American Healing Traditions, by Native American healer Helena Sheehan, Ph.D. Designed as a resource for health professionals, *Guided Imagery*, meticulously researched and authoritative, is essential reading for doctors, nurses, psychologists, counselors and all those involved or interested in healing.

CLOTH   400 PAGES   ISBN: 1899836446

"Well chosen, illuminating clinical examples abound, with eminently useful imagery suggestions for practitioner and patient."
—Belleruth Naparstek, LISW, author of *Staying Well with Guided Imagery*.

Also available: twin audiotape set of guided imagery scripts—
ISBN 1899836594 113 mins.

Instant Relaxation
How To Reduce Stress At Work, At Home
And In Your Daily Life
Debra Lederer & Michael Hall, Ph.D.

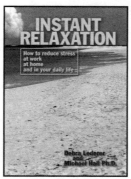

This is the last word in quick effective NLP and yoga techniques to reduce stress at work and at home. Debra has been utilizing and teaching these techniques for many years and sums them up as her state-of-the-art methods for "flying into a powerful and resourceful state of calm". The book offers a seven-day program of instruction into the methods, following which the reader will be able readily to access their relaxed core state. Michael Hall contributes by drawing on his vast knowledge of NLP to explain why Debra's methods are so powerful. Contents include: breath exercises, breath walking exercises, posture exercises, focused eye movements, affirmations, visualizations, pattern interrupts. Unlimited web support provided.

PAPER   136 PAGES   ISBN: 1899836365

"This is an exciting and innovative book. A masterpiece of its kind."
—*The Hypnotherapist*

Still – In The Storm
How To Manage Your Stress And
Achieve Balance In Life
Dr Ann Williamson

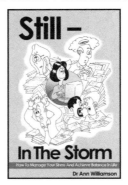

Why use this particular book to beat stress? Simple. This guide has been designed to be completely useable and accessible while at the same time presenting a program of exercises that will offer *long-term* stress solutions. It identifies and explains the most empowering, enjoyable and effective stress-relieving techniques, including: hypnosis, cognitive strategy, visualization, time management, relaxation, exercise, goal setting and positive mental rehearsal. Accessibility is the aim of this book – hence the clarity of its layout, its amusing cartoon illustrations and its reader-friendly tone. But as fun as it is, this book also offers a serious message and comes with the weighty assurance of its author's expertise: Dr Ann Williamson has no less than twenty-five years' experience of helping people handle anxiety.

PAPER   80 PAGES   ISBN: 1899836411

"A small but perfectly formed package of ideas to manage stress and achieve balance in life…. Genuinely amusing cartoons."
—*Time Out*

Vibrations For Health And Happiness
Everyone's Easy Guide To Stress-free Living
Tom Bolton

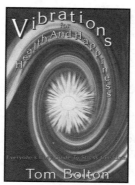

This is the first book ever to bring together, in one practical, accessible resource, all the information and techniques needed to relieve daily stress and tension, and attain optimum wholeness in life. A comprehensive guide and an exciting voyage into the world of holistic living, healing and wisdom, *Vibrations* ... enables the reader to see everything in a new light, filling their lives with health and happiness.

PAPER   248 PAGES   ISBN: 1899836160

"*Vibrations* ... is brilliant! It covers everything that anyone could ever need from a self-help book ... the most spiritually captivating book I have read for a long time."
—Betty Shine, author of *Mind Waves* and *Mind Magic*

USA & Canada *orders to:*

LPC Group
1436 West Randolph Street, Chicago, Illinois, 60607
Tel: 800-626-4330, Fax: 800-334-3892
www.lpcgroup.com

Australasia *orders to:*

Footprint Books Pty Ltd
Unit 4, 92A Mona Vale Rd, Mona Vale, NSW 2103, Australia
Tel: +61 2 9997 3973, Fax: +61 2 9997 3185
E-mail: info@footprint.com.au

UK & Rest of World *orders to:*

The Anglo American Book Company Ltd.
Crown Buildings, Bancyfelin, Carmarthen, Wales SA33 5ND
Tel: +44 (0)1267 211880/211886, Fax: +44 (0)1267 211882
E-mail: books@anglo-american.co.uk